Re-Imagining the End of Life:

Self-Development & Reflective Practices for Nurse Coaches

BY JANET BOOTH, MA, RN, NC-BC

THE WAY IT IS

THERE'S A THREAD YOU FOLLOW. IT GOES AMONG
THINGS THAT CHANGE. BUT IT DOESN'T CHANGE.
PEOPLE WONDER ABOUT WHAT YOU ARE PURSUING.
YOU HAVE TO EXPLAIN ABOUT THE THREAD.
BUT IT IS HARD FOR OTHERS TO SEE.
WHILE YOU HOLD IT YOU CAN'T GET LOST.
TRAGEDIES HAPPEN; PEOPLE GET HURT
OR DIE; AND YOU SUFFER AND GET OLD.
NOTHING YOU DO CAN STOP TIME'S UNFOLDING.
YOU DON'T EVER LET GO OF THE THREAD.

–William Stafford
Written 26 days before he died

Contents

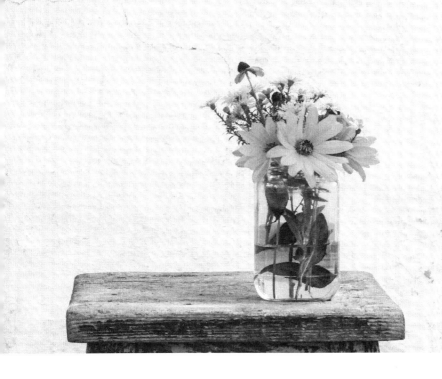

Acknowledgments

I am grateful to:

My supportive family and friends who have believed in me throughout this long process of distilling my passion for progressive end-of-life care into a concrete form – especially my loyal and encouraging husband, Bob.

The patients and families in hospice and palliative care settings who let me into their lives during a very tender time.

The thought-leaders who have inspired me over 5 decades of interest in end-of-life care.

My colleagues in nurse coaching who have encouraged me to find the intersection of nurse coaching and end-of-life advocacy.

The Goddard College faculty who worked with me -- with special thanks to the patient and skillful midwifing efforts of Caryn Mirriam-Goldberg.

And to Celeste Eizaguirre for her design skills and willingness to help make this book a reality.

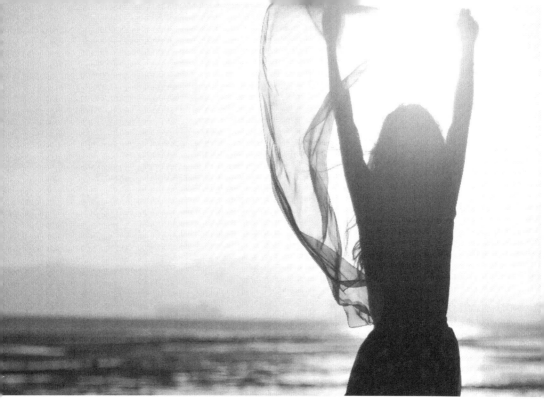

Introduction

THE ULTIMATE AIM OF NURSING AS A HUMAN CARING ART AND
SCIENCE IS TO ASSIST PERSONS AND SOCIETY IN BECOMING
MORE FULLY HUMAN.
(Lauterbach, 1996)

The purpose of this handbook is to provide you with opportunities for *reflection* and *inspiration* in your work as a nurse coach.

As nurses, many of us have seen firsthand that the process of navigating serious illness and death within our complex health care system is often confusing, isolating, crisis-driven, and dis-heartening.

What outcomes might be possible if

- we reimagined the end of life as a vital, purposeful stage of human development?

- practices of healing – forgiveness, gratitude, and letting go – became essential parts of our care plans?

- wisdom instead of fear informed our challenging decision points?

- we prepared for death in order to live more fully the time that we have?

- the hard work of caregiving was sustainable and meaningful for both family and professional caregivers?

Nurse coaching conversations involve presence, skillful listening, significant questions, reflection, and planning. They help guide individuals living with chronic and serious illness to make decisions about care and treatment within the framework of their own life story. By opening these conversations earlier in the trajectory of illness, we open the possibility of transforming how people experience the last part of their lives.

Our ability as nurse coaches to be compassionately present with people who are seriously ill and dying depends on our willingness to reflect on *our* own beliefs and worries about diminishment and mortality. This is how we "walk our talk."

In this handbook you will find tools and reflective practices that encourage you to explore your personal beliefs and values about aging, advanced illness, and dying. These practices will serve you well, both personally and professionally, for the rest of your life.

Sometimes, self-reflection on these topics stirs our emotions, brings back memories, or moves us from comfort to temporary discomfort. This is not a bad thing -- it's often a sign of stretching and growing our mind and spirit. I encourage you to trust yourself to move at your own pace with these reflective practices, and trust the process of exploring your human-ness.

The content of each chapter provides context for your exploration. What's the current landscape of end-of-life care, what is changing, and what might be possible? You may find fresh perspectives from thoughtful leaders in end-of-life care and a bigger picture of the emerging models in nursing and health care.

However, the real value of this handbook will come from your own reflections, writing, and sharing with others. You will find reflective practices at the end of each chapter, and a more extensive list of practices in Appendix D.

I encourage you to look for opportunities to share what you are exploring with the people closest to you. They will not only learn important information about you, but may also be inspired to do similar reflection and preparation.

Lastly, I hope this handbook will inspire you to reimagine the end of life as a vital part of how we become fully human – a time of life that holds value, meaning, and purpose. We see a significant cultural shift happening now with the emergence of new models for aging and dying. And, like any period of transition, such times can be confusing time for people to navigate and find their way.

The clarity and leadership of nurse coaches will help move us forward. Building that clear vision – and keeping it sustainable – depends on our willingness to do the inner work of self- development and self-care.

IT'S THE QUALITY OF YOUR APPROACH TO DYING THAT DETERMINES WHAT YOU'LL FIND.
–Stephen Jenkinson

There is a need for talking differently and more clearly about serious illness, dying, and grief. Who is going to take more leadership in these conversations? The shortage of trained palliative care nurses and other clinicians throughout the United States means that their expertise in goals-of-care conversations only benefits a relatively small percentage of seriously-ill people. And in spite of the importance of advance directives in dictating care, only about one-third of Americans have advance directives that outline their medical treatment wishes at the end of life (Yadav et al, 2017) – and only 25% of physicians know their patients have advance directives on file (CDC, 2012).

At the same time, there are people today who navigate advanced illness and dying with resiliency and psychosocial and spiritual wellbeing. They come to understand the positive potential of the end of life. There is much we can learn from them.

My own experience has convinced me that nurses and nurse coaches can contribute significantly to the transformation of end-of-life care in this country. As a nurse who has worked in end- of-life care for over thirty years, I have chosen to know dying. My initiation into the world of death and dying came suddenly during nursing school as an unexpected calling. I'd started nursing school with the intention of becoming a midwife and helping birth babies. But now I heard this new, clear call to serve instead as a midwife for the *dying*.

Since that time I have never looked back. My work trajectory has taken me from the bedside of hospice and palliative care patients to supporting the wellbeing of caregivers, and now into the larger community to further open our cultural conversation about end of life.

When people hear that I work in end-of-life care, some move away while others find me a safe place to tell their story. There are few places in American society where we speak openly of dying. For the last three decades I have been an end-of-life activist, guided by four simple beliefs whose roots have only deepened over time.

- We are all going to die someday.

- Death is a natural part of life.

- Most of us approach death unprepared for the journey ahead.

- Preparing for death can be one of the most healing and affirming acts of a lifetime.

One of the many lessons I learned at the bedside of dying people is how painful it is to come unprepared to the end of life, whether it is our own or that of our loved ones. Much of the suffering we experience seems to come from our *unfamiliarity* with the journey at end of life and our *not knowing* how to prepare for it. We lose track of where we are in the arc of our days and can easily become untethered from the thread of *what matters* most in our lives.

Preparation for dying, on the other hand, has the potential to affirm life and contribute to the healing of self and others. In my experience there is value in being *conscious* of how we live and die and more aware of the choices that may involve.

Coaching conversations help people honestly explore where they are, where they are heading, and how they want to get there. The coach's role in these conversations is partly to *guide* people through what may be foreign territory.

A guide is someone who is familiar with a place and leads travelers through new areas. She is able to communicate in a variety of languages and share her awareness of the culture of this new territory. She uses stories to bring the place to life and help others to see things they might not have noticed otherwise. A guide meets the travelers wherever they are, setting a tone of acceptance and hospitality that creates an atmosphere of trust. Perhaps most importantly, she assists the travelers in finding the confidence and resources they need to explore the territory on their own at some point.

The territory of aging, serious illness, and dying is not ordinary territory. It holds places most people don't want to go, or even talk about. It holds deep fears about being old, very sick, and dying. We may experience great suffering and isolation in these place as well as great peace and healing.

People often feel difficult emotions -- including loss, grief, and pain -- that most of us are unprepared to navigate. There are many stories to be told here, but we do not learn the language of these places until we find ourselves there.

This is no ordinary place, and yet it is a place of great humanity. Of human-making.

As a nurse coach, you have the opportunity to be on the forefront of a new model of humane health care – one that includes the promotion of wellbeing as well as advocacy for more compassionate end-of-life care.

- Nurse coaches focus on the wellbeing of the individual throughout the trajectory of chronic and advanced illness, and into the dying process.

- We work with people to make decisions and changes in their lives based on what matters most to them.

- We use high-level communication skills to open up conversations with people living with chronic and advanced illness.

- We draw on our depth of experience, skills, and knowledge to guide people in navigating the complex health care decisions and options at end of life.

Integrative Nurse Coaching

Most of my nursing career has been in end-of-life care (hospice and palliative care), but I have also maintained a secondary career in health and wellness promotion. While a student in the Integrative Nurse Coaching program (through the International Nurse Coach Association) in 2012, I envisioned bringing these two worlds together. When I shifted my focus from *wellness* to *wellbeing*, I saw how this new role of *nurse coach for people with serious illness* could serve as an innovative response to the crisis of how we die in the US. By becoming change agents in end-of-life advocacy work, nurses may also find an opportunity for greater leadership.

An integrative nurse coaching program covers three main areas of education and development for nurses: nurse coaching skills and practice, integrative nursing education and practice, and nurse self-development.

Nurse coach self-development is the first component of the theory that underpins integrative nurse coaching. It draws from the four areas of self-reflection, self-assessment, self-evaluation, and self-care. A core belief is that our ability to grow and develop as human beings is based on our willingness to engage with self-development throughout our lifetime.

Self-reflection also helps encourage a sense of *curiosity* and *care* in end-of-life work. Curiosity is a wonderful alternative to fear, especially when we are talking about scary and unfamiliar places. The *curiosity* starts with yourself and your own journey, and the *care* begins with yourself and your own wellbeing.

Reflection on our own beliefs and experiences increases our awareness, and this in turn builds our skills as reflective practitioners. Part of knowing the territory is knowing ourselves – having a spirit of curiosity about what's going on inside us. Taking time to reflect is key to understanding complex issues and challenges like the ones we face with serious illness and death. Reflecting on our own experiences with loss, grief, and dying can impact our care of people living with serious illness or at end of life. Reflecting purposely on our assumptions, biases, values, and beliefs can move us from habitual to more intentional action.

Care for yourself makes caring for others sustainable. Taking an assessment of our own health and wellbeing is a start. What positive health behaviors are already in place, and what additional practices might increase a sense of wellbeing and purpose? The practice of compassion and being fully present with others doesn't just happen – these skills can be learned and enhanced. We all need regular practices of health and wellbeing in order to have the stamina for the hard and rewarding work of caregiving.

At the heart of this handbook is an *exploration* of ideas...an *invitation* to reflect... and an *opportunity* to expand our conversations about living and dying. Through personal exploration we may discover what we bring to this conversation and what is ours to do next as advocates for quality end-of-life care.

Reflective Practices

1. Is there anything in your experience with seriously ill or dying patients that has troubled you? What weighs heavily on your heart? How have these feelings influenced your nursing practice?

2. Have you ever met someone who lived the last part of their life in a way that made you say, "That's how I want to do it!" What about that person's approach to living – and dying – affected you?

3. In her book, The Top 5 Regrets of the Dying, hospice nurse Bronnie Ware records the top five regrets of the dying people she cared for. Which of these regrets speak most to you? Why?

- I wish I'd had the courage to live a life true to myself, not the life others expected of me.

- I wish I hadn't worked so hard.

- I wish I'd had the courage to express my feelings.

- I wish I had stayed in touch with my friends.

- I wish that I had let myself be happier.

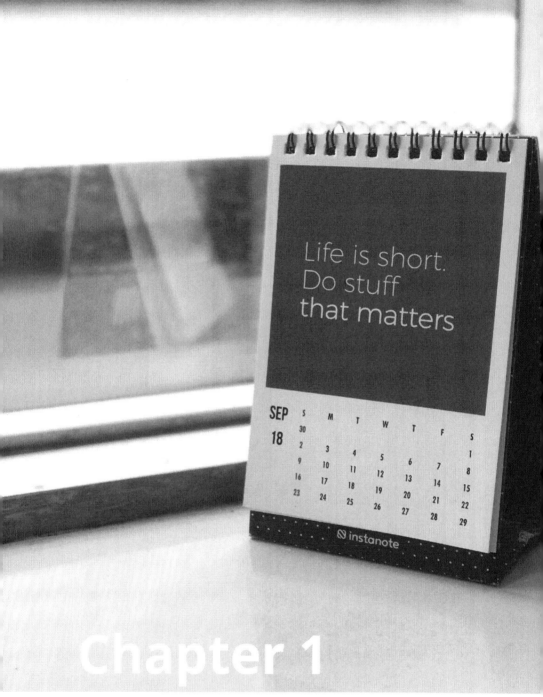

Chapter 1

The Nurse Coaching Model in End-of-Life Care

The Nurse Coaching Model in End-of-Life Care

The nurse coach model of practice is one of many ways that nurses have played a vital role as patient advocates and change agents within health care. Nurses have been on the forefront of many innovations in health care. Today we stand in a long line of nurse leaders and advocates – a proud lineage of nurses taking leadership in reforming health care. From Florence Nightingale to Dame Cecily Saunders, founder of the modern hospice movement, to Florence Wald, who started the first US hospice, and holistic nursing pioneer Barbara Dossey, we draw inspiration from the many nurses who have envisioned wellbeing in new, groundbreaking ways.

Included in these new approaches is the adoption of a coaching model into the work of integrative nursing. What is it about the integrative nurse coaching model that makes it so compatible with the complex experience of living with serious illness? Each component offers a special strength upon which to build our practice.

Integrative. We practice out of a model of care for the whole person – the bio-psychosocial-spiritual-cultural-environmental dimensions of health and wellbeing.

Nurse. Our clinical expertise includes an understanding of the science of the human body in both disease and health, and the daily health challenges with which many people live. Our grounding in the art of nursing emphasizes the values of caring, healing, trust, and compassion.

Coach. Our interactions are relationship-centered, results-oriented, and guided by the priorities and goals of the client.

Two of the co-creators of the integrative nurse coaching movement, Barbara

Dossey and Susan Luck, wrote in 2015:

Through the coaching relationship of trust and mutual respect, the Integrative Nurse Coach and client/patient are engaged in a manner that allows for a shift in consciousness and exploration of life's journey, health and wellbeing goals, and transformation.

For a person living with advanced illness, this exploration of health and wellbeing goals can be very helpful. It addresses priorities for the present while serving as a bridge to a potentially uncertain future.

I coached a woman with advanced cancer who was experiencing significant fatigue from both disease progression and medical treatment. She initially asked to problem-solve together what might reduce her fatigue and help her feel more energized. During our second session together, she remarked that it might not be reasonable to expect her old energy back; she knew that the cancer was spreading. In the next coaching conversation we then explored her priorities if her energy were to remain limited and she never regained her original baseline.

Often, people with serious illness are fighting to survive and at the same time hoping to return to former levels of health. An exploration of priorities for wellbeing in a time of increased diminishment can benefit patients by bringing them into the present. The questions for this woman became: How might she become more comfortable with things as they were? What did wellbeing look like today? What mattered most in her life, beyond the treatment of her disease?

This shift in focus significantly shaped her quality of life over the following months. She took her next steps forward based on the priorities that came out of our conversations. She told me later that it transformed how she lived each day. She was more present to herself and others, engaged more openly in conversations with her family, and found gratitude in places where she had previously felt worry or fear. This focus on a person's wellbeing can become a thread that continues through the spectrum of health, illness, and dying.

Patient-focused advocacy is a core competency for the professional nurse. We are frequently in a position to provide guidance for patients and families confronting difficult decisions and adapting to painful realities. Public opinion polls consistently rate nursing as the #1 most honest and ethical profession.

Some nurses feel comfortable and confident engaging openly with patients and families in challenging care conversations. However, multiple sources in nursing literature reveal barriers for nurses in leading these conversations about goals of care for people with serious illness. These barriers include discomfort, even fear, and educational deficiencies.

Discomfort and Fear

Over the past ten years, the three most frequently identified barriers to end-of-life advocacy by nurses in acute care were the physician, the patient's family, and fear (Hebert, Moore, Rooney, 2011). Nurses experienced fear as a barrier more often within hierarchical hospitals – for example, if nurses advocate for their patients, such as by sharing information about making informed decisions, conflict with the hospital administration may occur and result in disciplinary action (Thacker, 2008).

Nurses may also *hesitate to initiate conversations* out of fear of saying the wrong thing, fear of emotions (their own, the patient's, or the family's), and feelings of guilt because they aren't able to do more. They may disagree with the patient or the family's decisions for goals of care, leading to moral distress (Peereboom, Coyle, 2012).

Other obstacles to open conversations include perceptions that the patient or family members are unwilling to confront a terminal prognosis, the patient's inability to communicate, real or perceived physician reticence, and a desire to maintain hope of patients and family members (Peereboom, Coyle, 2012).

To address these issues, it is helpful for nurses to have honest and transparent advance care planning conversations with their *own* families and primary providers. By becoming more comfortable talking about dying with those they love and interact with most, nurses may become more comfortable talking about end-of-life care publicly (Giovanni, 2012).

Educational Deficiencies

Nurses can articulate the benefits of advance directives, but generally lack the knowledge and training to conduct such discussions with patients (Hebert, Moore, Rooney, 2011). It is important that nursing curricula include practice and mentoring in the area of end-of- life conversations, since proficiency in this type of communication will not be realized in the classroom alone (Giovanni, 2012). The End-of-Life Nursing Education Consortium (ELNEC) project is a good example of a national education initiative whose mission is to improve palliative care by educating nurses on better end-of-life care and communication. (See Appendix B for more information about the ELNEC program.)

Additionally, the cultural values and beliefs that inform bioethics practices in American hospitals and nursing school training tend to be white and middle class. Based on Western philosophical and legal traditions, they emphasize the individual and individual decision- making (Hebert, Moore, Rooney, 2011). The value of a team or family approach to end-of-life issues may be overlooked.

Benefits of the Nurse Coaching Model

In the world of serious illness and end-of-life care, the role of discussing goals of care with patients and families has traditionally been reserved for physicians. As nurses take more leadership in initiating these conversations, the coaching model provides a well-structured and purposeful approach.

Because nurses are highly trusted by patients and families, they have multiple opportunities in most practice settings to practice skillful questioning and deep listening with others. When people feel safe, heard, and respected, they are more likely to choose to explore their life's journey and share their vulnerabilities.

As the nurse coach builds on the person's strengths and confidence, a shift in thinking or feeling is more likely to happen. This positive momentum and human connection often encourages the person to move forward, which is especially helpful for those who feel stuck or fearful about change. People are more apt to make changes and decisions if they are based on their personal goals for wellbeing and peace of mind. All these steps contribute to the process of transformation from the old way to the new – to a reimagined way of living in the world.

These nurse coaching elements are consistent wherever our clients find themselves on the spectrum of living and dying. However, there are a few areas that might require more self- reflection and skillful, nuanced conversation with seriously ill people. One is our ability to *"hold space"* and be present with people who may be experiencing immediate and raw feelings of grief, loss, regret, or fear. It involves creating an environment that is safe, supportive, and non-judgmental. We must engage enough with our own fears and shadow emotions to be able to stay steady and compassionate when others fall apart. Frank Ostaseski, a thought- leader in compassionate presence for professional caregivers, has written:

> We can't travel with others in territory that we haven't explored ourselves. It's not often our expertise but the exploration of our own suffering that enables us to be of real assistance. That's what allows us to touch another human being's pain with compassion instead of with fear and pity. It is an intimacy with our own inner life that enables us to form an empathetic bridge to the other person (2008).

Calm, compassionate presence can create a sense of equanimity even when raw or complicated feelings are witnessed and held – without the need to label them as good or bad. This often encourages a sense of confidence that falling apart doesn't mean a person is permanently broken or lost. There is a way through these complex emotions. These are learned – and practiced – skills of a mindful nurse coach.

Another challenge is helping people explore **ambivalence** as they struggle with goals of care and medical decisions. A person may want to stop difficult treatments that aren't slowing disease progression *and* want to live as long as possible. Ambivalence is normal for most people when faced with change and transition, let alone loss. When a healthy person is ambivalent about health behavior changes, it might be easier for the nurse coach to remain detached and not try to argue for change – to "roll with the resistance." But when the stakes seem higher at end of life, and we as nurses understand the implications of choosing aggressive care or futile treatment, we may experience moral distress and feel unable to remain neutral and supportive. This is a place where the coaching techniques of Motivational Interviewing (MI) can provide support.

Ambivalence arises when there are two competing core values. Both values are important, and yet it's not clear which is the most important. When both sides of this ambivalence are explored, particularly through the use of reflective statements and summarizing, a person is better able to weigh the benefits and costs of the current situation. It brings the focus back to what matters most, which often helps to reduce a person's resistance and resolve the ambivalence. Working collaboratively to evoke a person's inner motivations helps that person to make decisions that are in alignment with their own values and goals, even if those are not necessarily the same as the nurse coach's (Pollak et al, 2011).

A third area that may require extra sensitivity and skill involves the complexity of a patient or family's **hope**. Many times, I've witnessed a shift along the continuum of illness from *hoping for cure to hoping for the best possible outcome*, which in turn might become for some *hope to not suffer at the end*. What complicates these shifts is the commonly held belief that to talk openly about the end of life is to give up hope. Hope for some people equals cure; for others, it's a significant source of strength and resilience that has gotten them to this point. What the nurse coach might offer instead is a broader definition of hope – what is the best quality of life to hope for at this point in a person's life, and what matters most? For some people, it can be helpful to frame the conversation as "What would you want to happen if things don't turn out the way you hope?" Conversations about quality of life throughout the course of aging and illness can become another thread that guides people's decisions in a meaningful way. Skillful questions, deep listening, and compassionate presence serve nurse coaches well as they explore these sensitive areas with patients and families.

As seen with the use of the word "hope," language can be a powerful tool. It has the potential either to open up or to shut down conversations. As nurse coaches, it's wise to reflect on the words and communication styles we use habitually – and how our communication might create unnecessary barriers to authentic conversation.

What routine phrases or explanations do we offer without much thought ("a good death," "he failed treatment," "she's non-compliant," "they're in denial")? What assumptions do we make about other peoples' values and beliefs? As patient advocates and "translators" of information, nurses are typically on the forefront of effective health communication with patients. In discussions of goals of care and end-of-life decision-making with patients and families with low *health literacy*, we often see less advance directive completion and less certainty about available choices. In the acute setting, health care providers may ask for decisions that are hurried, or patients may have limited understanding of the choices they are making. Patients may be confused by language, the variety of people involved in their care, and the expectations of the hospital culture. It's helpful to slow down our speech, speak in shorter chunks of information, check frequently for comprehension, and involve surrogates or family members who are trusted by the patient.

Terminology also becomes complex at end of life due to the reluctance of many practitioners to use words like "dying" or "terminal illness." Many patients and families are reluctant to speak of death. Euphemisms are used, which by nature are not specific or clear. Hard truths are masked by hopeful comments, perhaps out of a desire to protect people from pain, but most likely only kicking the hard decisions further down the road. It's further complicated in health care settings when the professionals having the hard conversations aren't necessarily known or trusted by the patient and family. How do we as health care clinicians acknowledge the time of dying – actually recognize and name it – when we might know little about the people in front of us? How do we speak and act in a way that encourages trust in this vulnerable time?

In our first encounter with a patient, we may have to overcome an initial attitude of *mistrust* on the part of the patient or family. This is particularly true when talking about withdrawing treatments or initiating a DNR order for people with a history of systemic inequality and lack of access to care, such as African Americans and Latinos. Justin Sanders, a physician at Dana Farber Cancer Center, writes:

> In order for health literacy to emerge in a way that supports advance care planning and palliative care, we must focus not on advance directives...but on scalable, translatable communication practices that help patients and clinicians enter an inevitable space together, arm-in-arm, without fear of ineptitude (clinicians) or abandonment (patients).

Conversations that focus on procedures will never be effective on their own with certain populations because they are hard to understand and they prioritize the clinician's goals, not the patient's (2015).

These communication practices that Sanders refers to fit well in the context of a coaching conversation that is relationship-based, patient-focused, and collaborative. It takes skill and courage for a clinician to enter that "inevitable space" alongside the patient, and to acknowledge that they are all in a place of *not-knowing* the answer. Only then does the exploration together allow decisions about care and treatments for the patient to arise out of the values and meaning of the patient's own life story.

Nurse coaches also participate collaboratively in complex situations through the practice of *cultural competency*. This is the traditional concept of becoming aware of cultural differences (particularly with vulnerable populations) and how our biases or assumptions might affect our work as health care providers. Such cultural self-reflection is especially important when navigating the complexities of health care at the end of life. A further step in understanding cultural differences is the experience of *cultural humility*, which aligns well with the coaching perspective. Silvia Austerlic, the Latino Community Liaison for the Hospice Caring Project in California, describes cultural humility as

> the complex attitude and sensitive skills required to meet the needs of patients and families in a way that empowers them to participate in a two-way therapeutic relationship, where both patient and provider are understood to have something to contribute (2009).

This process requires us as health care providers to willingly suspend our beliefs in order to hear more clearly what matters most to patients and their families. A patient or family's cultural norms may be quite different from our own. For example, the core American values of autonomy and an individual's right to make life choices may not be the priority values of our patients or their families. As a strong advocate for conscious end-of-life care choices, I have found this challenging at times. It has opened my mind to other ways of achieving the best possible care in dying that are right for someone else.

When are people most open to conversations about end of life priorities? Often, transition points in a person's illness offer the best opportunities for coaching conversations. These are times to revisit what's happening, what are the priorities and goals of care, and what resources might be needed. The structure and "next steps" focus of the coaching model can be reassuring for the patient and family. Karen Peereboom and Nessa Coyle have written about useful language in goals of care discussions. (Their approach is similar to a coaching model – you can find their chart of helpful questions in Appendix B. You may be interested as well in the structure of the *Serious Illness Conversation Guide*, also found in Appendix B.)

Identifying the goals of a particular patient and helping them to reach goals may include their need to reframe or modify the goal as life draws to an end. This is an extremely important nursing role. The ability to sit with the patient and hear his/ her grief as losses accumulate, goals are modified, and hope redefined is integral to communication in nursing care at the end of life (Peereboom, Coyle, 2012).

Finding the appropriate language and open-ended questions that can help reframe a goal is part of the work of nurse coaches. At the center of this high-level communication, however is sitting with the person – listening, and in silence.

The structure and shape of each coaching conversation may differ, depending on the practice setting and the needs of the person being coached. Nurse coaches work within hospital settings, in primary care practices, in community organizations, and in independent practice. Sometimes individual sessions are best, while other times group coaching models are effective for families or communities. Sometimes time constraints allow only "laser coaching" of 5-10 minutes, while other times a nurse coach may have 45-60 minutes to work with people. In addition to the goals of care conversations, coaching sessions might focus on other priorities a person has for their life: getting financial and legal paperwork in order, scheduling time with family and friends, or organizing a legacy project. Nurse coaches can make a big difference in the lives of caregivers, whether family or professional, by helping them to create a do-able, achievable plan of wellbeing and resilience practices. Additionally, some nurse coaches have found a niche in working with people who are experiencing grief, loss, and bereavement. There are many different ways to help transform serious illness and end-of-life care as a nurse coach.

When we engage as nurse coaches in conversations with people about end-of-life care, we are talking about much more than their symptoms and treatment choices. We are addressing the whole person, in the context of their family and their culture. And we are with them in some of the most difficult and troublesome times of their lives. Patients may be adjusting to a life completely changed after a terminal diagnosis, or navigating one loss after another as they imagine the end of their life. Family members and friends are managing their own difficult emotions of pain, loss, and perhaps fear. What we bring into those moments may be the best medicine we can offer – presence, attention, caring, and a willingness to bear witness to their experience. These sensitive, deeper skills of communication within the nurse coaching model reflect the healing that is possible within the complicated landscape of care at the end of life.

Reflective Practices

1. Watch this seven-minute clip from the movie, Wit.
https://www.youtube.com/watch?v=RS8Bqgie_RA

The nurse (Susie) is caring for a woman (Vivian) with end-stage cancer who is trying to decide about her DNR status.

- What was most important to each of the characters in this scene?

- What stood out to you in their interaction?

- Was there anything that made you uncomfortable?

2. Consider the contrasting beliefs below. Note which one you value more. Give a strong argument for the opposite belief, and how it could have equal value to your own.

- Mourning a death openly vs. projecting stoicism

- Life support should be used whenever possible vs. allow a natural death

- Death is the end vs. there is life after death

- A person should be told they are dying vs. a person should not be told they are dying

- A person has the right to state their own end of life wishes vs. the family unit should decide end of life care.

3. What do you think happens when we die? How did you arrive at those ideas or beliefs?

4. In your last days...

- Where do you want to die, and why?

- What would the last week or day of your life look like?

- How will the space around your bedside look, sound, smell, and feel?

- Who would you like to be there?

- Who would you not want to be there?

- How do you want people to interact with you and talk to you?

- What people and/or animals do you want present for your last breath?

- What do you want done with your body after you die?

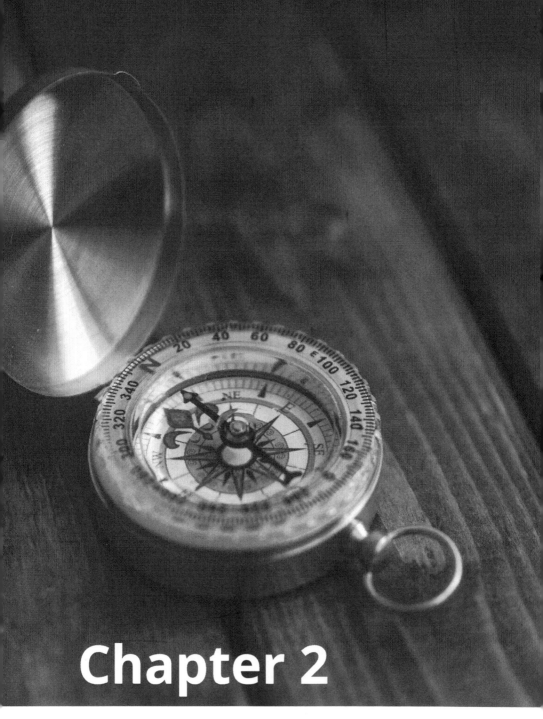

Chapter 2

Where Are We? Locating Ourselves in the Landscape of End-of-Life Care

Where Are We? Locating Ourselves in the Landscape of End-of-Life Care

When my father was growing up in small towns in Maine in the 1920s and 1930s, most people died at home. To see aging and dying up close was not unusual, whether it was grandparents living with the family or young people helping with the tasks of caregiving. More of the population in rural communities had exposure to animal deaths and the cycles of nature, and the local community attended at-home viewings and funerals. At that time there weren't enough doctors or effective medicines, and most people died from relatively simply infections. When medical advances became available to prolong life and fight disease, this was seen as a very good thing. Infections could be treated, stopped hearts re-started, failing kidneys sustained, cancers imaged by machines, and insulin supplemented with a simple injection. The place we find ourselves now, 80 years later, is a very different landscape. Most people are doing the best they can to navigate the *unintended consequences* of these many medical-technological advances.

My experience is that most people living with chronic and advanced illness want quality of life as a goal of care, but they don't always know how to operationalize that within the health care system. To better understand this landscape of modern end-of-life care, let's look at *four key influences* that impact our experiences:

- the nature of modern disease,

- the first wave of innovative practices,

- roadblocks to open conversations, and

- the redefinition of dying well.

The nature of modern disease

One of the most significant consequences of this new landscape of medical science is that death is often seen as a *failure* of medicine. So many improvements were made, both in the treatment of chronic disease and in extending longevity, that it appeared as if we could hold off death. In the past, Uncle Joe's diabetes and high blood pressure might have led to irreparable damage and death by the time he was 50. Now, Uncle Joe may live into his 80s, but he is on a slow decline that includes numerous hospitalizations and a questionable quality of life. We are unlikely to say that Uncle Joe is dying. Instead, we say he's chronically ill or disabled, needs more nursing care or even formal medical supervision as he experiences failing health.

In the past, it was easier to see patterns of weakness and disability in people who were old or very sick. There was a familiarity with such decline that came from multiple generations living together, or from close proximity to neighboring families. It was expected that someone with an infection or significant trauma to the body would likely die – and most people could probably recognize the signs of dying. In modern times, however, people often wait for experts within the healthcare system to tell them that they're dying. The expectation now is that medical science can reverse the course of dying much of the time. This creates a wide array of options and a momentum towards cure and *not-dying*.

When do we shift our treatment focus from *living with* serious illness to *dying from* serious illness? This shift in focus will impact how people make medical decisions, who decides their goals of care, and the timing of when these discussions occur. The lack of clarity between *living with* and *dying from* illness can result in confusion, regret, and even moral distress for some people as they try to find their way through these unfamiliar places at end of life.

Current statistics show that most Americans will live with at least one chronic disease as they age, and die slowly from progressive or advanced disease. Most of us will have lots of time to prepare. One way to orient ourselves to the experience of living with advanced illness is to talk about *disease trajectory*, or what we might expect in the course of any particular disease process. People with a similar diagnosis have unique courses of disease, and yet there are patterns of diminishment and deterioration that are shared and predictable. Health care providers can help the patient and family to understand the patient's medical and functional condition, and what that might look like over the months or years ahead. They can try to anticipate events that will likely occur. The goal of these conversations about advanced illness is to be more proactive in making decisions, and to have those decisions made in the context of a patient's goals and values, rather than simply reacting to changes in condition.

The trajectories of how we die have actually changed a lot over the past 50 years. There are now three main trajectories at end of life: the more precipitous decline of end-stage cancer; the slow downward curve – and occasional crises – of end-stage disease and chronic illness; and the slow and steady decline of dementia and Alzheimer's (Murray, Kendall, et al, 2005). There are expected points along these trajectories where honest assessments and transparent conversations about goals of care could beneficially occur.

For example, the first trajectory features a short period of evident decline, as typically seen with cancers. We see weight loss, decreased performance status, and reduced self-care – and then a precipitous drop in function. Along the second trajectory – as seen with end-stage heart, lung, or kidney diseases – we see long-term limitations develop through intermittent serious episodes and a declining baseline. Deterioration is usually associated with admission to the hospital, often the emergency room or intensive care unit, and the person's baseline functioning never regains pre-hospital status. The third typical trajectory of progressive disease can be described as "prolonged dwindling," as in the case of end-stage brain diseases such as dementias and Alzheimer's. It includes multi-system frailty: the baseline functioning is low, accompanied by increasing, progressive disability.

These trajectories all have expected crises and decision-points attached to them. As people better understand what is a typical progression towards end of life, they often have opportunities to make conscious decisions about treatment and how they want to live out the end of their days. As discussed in Chapter 1, these major transition points are a natural time to revisit goals of care and what matters most to patients and families. These points include:

- When signs and symptoms point to further disease progression
- When functional decline affects quality of life
- When treatments might start causing more harm than benefit.

It's not surprising that many people are unfamiliar with these transition points and how they fit into the context of natural, inevitable aging and dying. Throughout the last part of the 20th century, aging and dying were increasingly "out-sourced" to institutions or professionals through the growth of nursing homes, hospitals, and funeral homes. This outsourcing was accompanied by a subsequent decrease in family and community involvement with the realities of death and dying. With increased economic opportunity for many people, fewer extended families lived together and more women joined the workforce. These changes had an impact on families' ability to give care to aging and ill members. Without a community context for witnessing and discussing how we die, many people became detached from the experience and language of serious illness and dying, such as caregiving,

14

reviewing one's life and legacy, after-death care, and grief and bereavement. The social fabric that holds this part of our human story together has shifted, bringing both crisis and opportunity.

First-wave innovative practices

Over the past 50 years, various thought-leaders and innovators who understood the unintended consequences of modern disease treatment saw an opportunity to create more clear and compassionate models for dying. The initial wave of end-of-life innovation and change came in the 1960s and 1970s. These new initiatives were responsible for re-directing the trajectory of end-of-life care. Four central innovations centered around Elizabeth Kubler Ross' groundbreaking book, *On Death and Dying*; the modern hospice movement; the creation of palliative care; and the introduction of advance directives.

Kubler-Ross' book was a countercultural phenomenon that spoke with candor and fierceness about people dying in isolation and pain. It opened a new conversation about death by telling the stories of those who were dying, and bringing the reader right into that experience.

> Those who have the strength and the love to sit with a dying patient in the *silence that goes beyond words* will know that this moment is neither frightening nor painful, but a peaceful cessation of the functioning of the body. Watching a peaceful death of a human being reminds us of a falling star; one of the million lights in a vast sky that flares up for a brief moment only to disappear into the endless night forever (Kubler-Ross, 1969).

The first hospice in the US, founded in 1974, provided a model for the kind of peaceful death that Kubler-Ross imagined. Hospice showed people how to care for people at the end of life at home, with family caregivers supported by a skilled interdisciplinary heath care team, and a holistic approach to alleviating pain and suffering. It's instructive to note that after 40 years of hospice in our country – and very high marks from consumers who are grateful for the services – the median length of stay in hospice programs is still only one to two weeks. Given that most people die slowly from one or more chronic and serious illnesses, such short hospice stays speak to a real ambivalence about shifting from curative to palliative care in the last part of our lives.

Palliative care services developed in the 1990s and draw from the same central elements of hospice care, but are made available to patients and families throughout the whole trajectory of illness. Most major hospital systems have palliative care teams who are brought in as consultants for their expertise in both pain/symptom management and complex, sensitive discussion about goals of care. The development of hospice and palliative care was a direct response to the medicalized approach to dying that had inadvertently created a new set of challenges for how we die. These movements changed the landscape of serious illness, dying, and death in favor of open conversation, compassion, and whole-person care.

Life-extending treatments also create situations where people may be kept alive despite poor quality of life. The cases of Karen Anne Quinlan (1976), Nancy Cruzan (1990), and Terry Schiavo (2005) – all of whom lived in a "persistent vegetative state" without clear end-of-life wishes – brought national attention to these issues. Advance directives were developed as an essential legal document that assures the right of an individual to refuse medical treatment and to have those wishes respected even if the dying person is unable to communicate. Today, the default in our medical system is aggressive care unless there is a clearly written advance directive that has been communicated clearly to the health care team. However, only about one-third of adults have completed an advance directive. Contributing factors include lack of awareness or denial of the need for an advance directive and its importance, confusion and ambivalence about end-of-life decisions, and cultural differences in navigating end-of-life care.

Roadblocks to open conversations

The need for change and further evolution in end-of-life care has been echoed at the national level by many organizations. The Institute of Medicine released *Dying in America: Improving Quality and Honoring Individual Preferences Near the End of Life*, a 2014 report that called for major reform of end-of-life care. The authors stated clearly that comprehensive care should

- be integrated, patient-centered, family-oriented;

- consider the evolving physical, emotional, social, and spiritual needs of individuals approaching the end of life, as well as those of their family and/or caregivers;

- be consistent with individuals' values, goals, and informed preferences.

They also concluded that dying in America is still harder than it needs to be – and that it is time for conversations about dying to become part of everyday life.

What gets in the way of these more open, intentional conversations recommended by the Institute of Medicine and many others? As already noted, death and dying are generally considered taboo as discussion topics, and death is often perceived as a failure of medicine. Our complex health care system makes it challenging to carry out thoughtful conversations with patients and families. Appointments are fast-paced and practitioners often hurried. Inter-professional communication and collaboration is often lacking. The language we use with patients is not always understood, or may not be culturally sensitive. Another key failure is that most health care practitioners are uncomfortable having sensitive conversations about preparation for dying, let alone facing their own fears and worries about diminishment and mortality.

It seems natural to us to be uncomfortable, anxious, or fearful about the fact of death. In my experience, out of all the thoughts and emotions we experience about end of life, nothing quite holds the place of *fear* as a barrier to reflection and conversation. There are potentially a multitude of fears at play as we contemplate dying and death, whether it is our own or another's: fear of the unknown, of pain or suffering, of not existing, of judgment or hell, of loss of identity and relationships. We fear grief, deep sadness, and anguish...separation from those we love...losing control or dignity or status...being a burden to others...leaving loved ones behind. There's also the fear of never having really lived, or having taken life for granted. These complex feeling are not easy to sit with and contemplate, and for that reason are often not something we can make peace with *at the last minute*.

An essential piece of this "inner work" at end of life – as throughout the whole of our life – might be to find a healthy response to feelings of emotional and spiritual *pain*. It may show up as unease, discomfort, or fear, but it is still related to pain. Most of us growing up didn't learn skills for coping with feelings of pain. In fact, we might say Americans are experiencing an epidemic of "numbing" ourselves to pain and stress by means of alcohol and opioid abuse, overuse of internet and television, overwork, overeating, and living in hectic overdrive.

I have seen tools of reflection and self-awareness help many people better understand their emotions of pain and loss. These tools help us to navigate the "groundlessness" – the feeling that the rug has been pulled out from under us – that arises, for example, when we are confronted with a new diagnosis of advanced illness. This sudden awareness of our vulnerability is threatening, and the existential suffering that results is often unfamiliar territory. Learning to live in this place with greater wellbeing requires us to find meaning and a kind of peace that will carry us through even the most heavy, stressful times. (One of the most effective tools to enhance wellbeing that nurse coaches learn is the practice of *mindfulness* – paying attention purposefully to what's happening in the present moment in our body, mind, and spirit. More on that in Chapter 4.)

Redefinition of dying well

As we further explore wellbeing at the end of life – the qualities of *dying well* – it helps to hear what others have said they wanted. The express wishes of the dying may help us reshape the modern redefinition of dying well. Recently, the *American Journal of Geriatric Psychiatry* made a list of ten core themes associated with dying well, culled from interviews and research in 36 studies (Meier et al, 2016).

1. Having control over the specific dying process

2. Pain-free status

3. Engagement with religion or spirituality

4. Experiencing emotional well-being

5. Having a sense of life completion or legacy

6. Having a choice in treatment preferences

7. Experiencing dignity in the dying process

8. Having family present and saying goodbye

9. Quality of life during the dying process

10. A good relationship with healthcare providers

Note that the majority of these wishes relate to psycho-spiritual wellbeing and relationships. This is where many people hope to arrive at the end of their lives. How might nurse coaches support people in planning ahead for these outcomes, and leading them to develop a deeper understanding of the positive potential at the end of life?

The core themes of *dying well* also help us to identify three basic categories of what matters most to people in medical decision-making: 1) quality vs. quantity of life; 2) the benefit vs. burden of treatments; 3) control vs. lack of control throughout the process. The weighing of these competing values, which often show up as *ambivalence*, offers a potent area for discussion with patients and families when discerning direction and priorities at end of life. Where does a person find themselves along the spectrum of those values? For example, patients and families may need to make hard decisions about life-sustaining treatments such as cardiopulmonary resuscitation, intubation and mechanical ventilation, artificial hydration, feeding tubes, antibiotics, or dialysis. Each treatment decision is challenging when the likelihood of recovery is unclear. There is no one choice that is obviously the right one – the context is instead a *gray area*. The benefits vs. burdens of these treatments need to be weighed carefully, bringing to bear both medical information and the patient's wishes. Will this treatment improve quality of life, restore function, and reduce pain and suffering, or will it lead to the opposite outcome? What has the patient written or expressed verbally in the past about their wishes at end of life? What are the highest priorities for this person?

Nurse coaches use their skills and sensitivities to illuminate such gray areas for patients and their families. Recently, the American Nurses Association (ANA) published a position statement on *Nurses' Roles and Responsibilities in Providing Care and Support at the End of Life* (2016). It stresses the importance of nursing leadership in conversations with patient and families about end-of-life care.

> Decision-making for the end of a patient's life should occur over years rather than just in the minutes or days before a patient's death. Nurses can be a resource and support for patients and families at the end of a patient's life and in the decision- making process that precedes it. Nurses are often ideally positioned to contribute to conversations about end-of-life care and decisions, including maintaining a focus on patients' preferences, and to establish mechanisms to respect the patient's autonomy.

This clear directive from the ANA helps nurses place themselves as key practitioners within the continuity of end-of-life care. We are encouraged to hold clarifying conversations with our patients over time, throughout the trajectories of illness. Nurse coaches can play an important role in helping to shift a person's experience away from the immediate crisis and toward the bigger picture of "what matters most." This shift requires a kind of pause, an opening, a relaxing, a chance to breathe more easily as patients and families reflect and re- calibrate the path forward. It allows us to find ourselves – to locate ourselves again – in the shifting landscape of serious illness and end of life.

Discussions of advance directives and decision points are part of a larger coaching conversation that is possible only when we take the long view of what guides us in life. This longer view entails a sense of continuity that allows us to make decisions and choose directions in the context of that which we value most. Physician Atul Gawande, author of *Being Mortal* (2014), writes,

> Our reluctance to honestly examine the experience of aging and dying has increased the harm we inflict on people and denied them the basic comforts they most need. Lacking a *coherent view* of how people might live successfully all the way to their very end, we have allowed our fates to be controlled by the imperatives of medicine, technology, and strangers.

Rather than coherence (understood as "the quality of forming a unified whole"), our medical approach to dying has been more narrowly focused on "not dying." Over the past 70 years advances in medical technology have led to great improvements in health care, especially in acute and emergent care. However, an unintended consequence of this life-saving imperative is that many people no longer know the place of natural death. Increasingly, people are asking for a more whole-person, developmental approach to the last part of our lives – a sense that dying fits into the unified whole of who we are, of the cycle of our life. A "coherent view" includes end of life as a *valuable developmental stage* with its own possibilities for healing, purpose, and wellbeing.

Reflective Practices

1. Locate a copy of the document *5 Wishes (fivewishes.org/five-wishes)* and fill it out, if you haven't already. Was there anything that surprised you in your responses? What was the hardest part to fill out?

2. Schedule a meeting or conversation with the person you've designated as your medical power of attorney. Review what is included in your wishes – the "law" of your advance directives. Then try to express more of the "spirit" of your wishes. What values and priorities are most important to you in the event that someone needs to make decisions on your behalf?

3. What am I most afraid of in getting older? What do I fear most about living with advanced illness? What really scares me about dying or about death? What is at the heart of those fears?

4. A Significant Loss. Think about the deaths you have experienced in your life, and choose one involving a person close to you. Let yourself connect as deeply as you can with the feelings, images, sounds, and events surrounding this death. The closer you get to the experience of that death, the more meaning you can pull out of the loss – and the greater your understanding of how it has shaped your thoughts about dying and death.

- Who died?

- What was their relationship to you?

- What was the cause of death?

- How long was the person sick?

- When did they die?

- How were you involved with the person as he or she was dying?

- Write about 2-3 moments or experiences during the dying process that stand out in your mind, both positive and negative. Why are these events important to you?

- What images, sounds, smells, or things said (or not said) in this person's last hours and days keep coming back into your mind after the death?

- How did your experience with this death confirm or change your thinking about what makes a "good" death and what happens afterwards?

- What did you learn about "being present" and caring for someone who is dying? As you look back now, what do you wish had been different?

- How did this death impact your life?

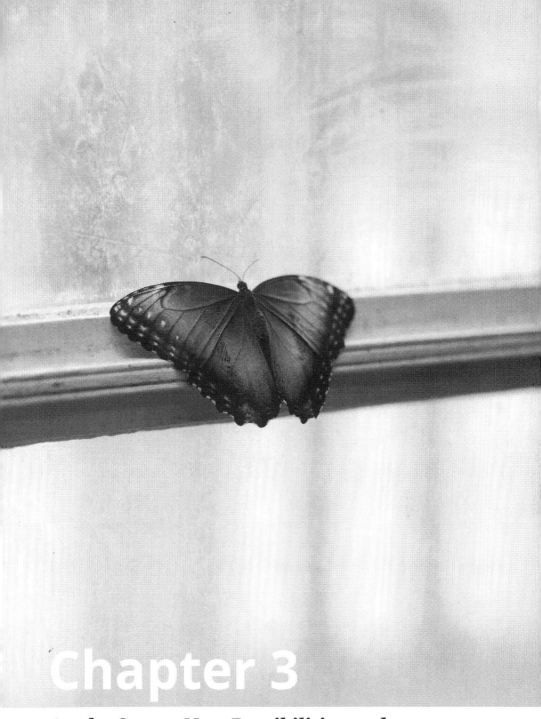

Chapter 3

*On the Cusp – New Possibilities and
Emerging Models*

AS LIVING HUMAN BEINGS, THE MOST REWARDING PURPOSE
OF OUR LIVES IS TO AWAKEN TO OUR DEEPEST REALITY,
TO UNFOLD OUR MOST POWERFUL ENERGIES OF LOVE AND
COMPASSION. THE STUDY OF AND PREPARATION FOR DEATH
MAY BE THE GREATEST OPPORTUNITY TOWARDS LEARNING TO
LIVE A FULLER LIFE.

– Robert Thurman

On the Cusp – New possibilities and emerging models

Albert Einstein reminds us that we can't solve our problems with the same thinking that got us into them. In the case of modern end-of-life care, death isn't the problem. Our response of *denial* to the reality of death is the problem that causes much suffering. How might nurse coaches help people find their way to a different way of being with death and dying? As stated in the Introduction to this handbook,

> A guide is someone who is familiar with a place and leads travelers through new areas. She is able to communicate in a variety of languages and share her awareness of the culture of this new territory. She uses stories to bring the place to life and help others to see things they might not have noticed otherwise.

To imagine new possibilities, we as nurse coaches might benefit by drawing from a different well of thinking and experience – a different kind of *knowing*, perhaps, and with a sense of curiosity. Part of the exploration in this chapter is based on a more mythic understanding of the meaning of living and dying, and the mysteries connected with our transition from this physical life to what may come next. Such an approach may help correct the imbalance that results from relying exclusively on a rational, scientific, biomedical model of dying, and *change the conversation* we're having about the end of life. This chapter is an invitation to explore a larger vision of aging and dying, and to imagine death as part of living a fuller life.

Author Michael Meade, who studies myth and storytelling, describes the ancient Greek conception of two ways of accounting for what happens in the world – and to us, as individuals in the world. *Logos* is all about logic and a linear timeline, and is very familiar to us in the modern Western world. Facts tell the whole story and can explain most everything. *Mythos* is a different kind of knowing that is narrative-based, rather than logic-based. It concerns story, not facts, and the deep subjective feelings a person has about life and death. It explores meaning, mystery, intuition, and the "dream hidden inside our lives," going beyond facts such as how old we are and what we look like. Mythos is about emotion and, most of all, *imagination*.

> If the power of logos is thinking in a logical way, the power of mythos is imagining. Mythos is the way in which our imagination re-organizes the world into a story that includes us in the story of the world (Living Myth, Episode 1 podcast, 2016)

What do aging, illness, and dying look like through the lens of mythos? The answer requires a shift in our thought process, our consciousness, as we move from a familiar way of thinking and acting to a new way. How might this shift help us reimagine the possibilities for our lives? The nurse coach's work is to ask open-ended questions, listen deeply, and allow space for a person's exploration of thoughts and feelings. We listen without judgment to another person's beliefs and values, psychospiritual experiences, inner wisdom, and intuition, and to their priorities for the next chapter of their life story. This more intentional and imaginative approach is one of the innovations emerging in end-of-life care.

Re-imagining end-of-life care involves creative thinking and seeing beyond the current dominant medical narrative about dying. It asks us to reflect and remain open to new ideas. When our culture goes too far in one direction, there is a natural correction that occurs – we move from death in isolation towards death within a community, from death as taboo towards more open conversations about dying, and from death as failure towards death as a natural part of being human. Out of the biomedical model of dying is emerging a bigger vision that includes a more holistic perspective. It's big enough to hold both science and spirit, matter and consciousness, health and healing, the individual and the community. And there's room for both the facts of dying and the unfolding *story* of our dying.

What do some of the leading theorists of human growth and development have to say about the last part of our lives? Erik Erikson names the core theme of our time between age 65 to death as *ego integrity vs. despair*. Ego integrity speaks to wholeness, as life review leads us to the culmination of life wisdom. The task here is *retrospection*, looking at the whole of our lives. Looking back on their lives, people may feel contentment, a sense of wholeness, completion, or integrity, or they may feel a sense of despair over not having lived their lives as they had hoped and intended (Miller, 2009). Carl Jung writes poetically of the "autumn of our lives" as an *inward* journey. He envisions life as a continuous search for the true self, with its second half a time for self-exploration and a discovery of meaning.

> A human being would certainly not grow to be seventy or eighty years old if this longevity had no meaning for the species. The *afternoon of life* must have a significance of its own and cannot be merely a pitiful appendage of life's morning (1957).

Lars Tornstam's *gerotranscendence theory* builds on Jung's perspective. This theory explains aging from a psychosocial perspective, and offers a developmental model of positive aging. It reflects the shift in the last part of our lives to a deepening wisdom and spirituality, a decreased fear of death, and an increased sense of intergenerational continuity. "Positively aging adults" are more able to counterbalance the inevitable losses of the aging process by focusing on what is important in life (2011). With most people in the US living into their 80s, we now spend a significant amount of time in this stage of development. It's not meant to be a holding space or a parking spot, but rather a time of life with its own intelligence and purpose.

One effective way to engage in conversations about end-of-life wishes is by asking the question of what it means to "age well." Talking about the challenges and opportunities inherent in aging is a meaningful segue for many people to the challenges and opportunities at the end of life. Tornstam's approach gives us a container big enough to include both positive aging *and* a preparation for dying – an approach that transcends the duality of living and dying. We find room for preparing to die within the context of living fully. In fact, there is value in considering these dimensions of life together – they enhance each other. In an American culture that values independence, youth, and productivity, we can draw upon another model that speaks to the value of older people who have slowed down and yet contribute in a different way to society. Although the role of elders has been lost in many parts of American society, there is a strong undercurrent occurring to revitalize the value and service of elderhood in our communities.

Notice how the threads of *healing, wisdom,* and *wellbeing* are interwoven throughout the theories outlined above. These qualities are at the heart of our practice as nurse coaches. There are many ways to define these concepts. For the purposes of this handbook, here are some helpful ways to define these terms.

> *Healing* is a shift in quality of life away from anguish and suffering, toward an experience of integrity, wholeness, and inner peace. This shift in quality of life is the overarching goal of whole person care... (Hutchinson, 2011).

> *Wisdom* involves an integration of knowledge, experience,

and deep understanding that incorporates tolerance for the uncertainties of life, as well as its ups and downs (Psychology Today blog, 2017).

Wellbeing is a general term for the condition of an individual or group and their social, economic, psychological, spiritual, or medical state; based on the idea that the way each person thinks and feels about her or his life is meaningful and important (Dossey et al, 2015).

In the lives of older people we see possibilities for healing when there's no cure, for sharing wisdom instead of productivity, and for wellbeing in the midst of serious illness. This shift in perspective is significant. Nurse coaches have the potential to change lives by exploring these concepts with people who may feel diminished, marginalized, or without purpose. This process can lead to a place of profound re-imagining. Ira Byock, a palliative care physician, acknowledges the significance of this shift in perspective when he writes

Understanding how individuals approaching death are able to transition from experiencing a sense of meaninglessness and impending annihilation to a sense of wholeness and "wellness" has profound practical implications...If a sense of impending disintegration and the loss of meaning underlie suffering, it is not surprising that a sense of well-being involves a preserved – or enhanced – sense of integrity and meaning (2016).

This transition from meaninglessness to meaning, from disintegration to integration, is a process that can be nurtured and developed. Coaching conversations that include aspects of life review and life completion have been shown to improve a sense of wellbeing for seriously ill people (Steinhauser, Alexander, Byock, 2009). I've heard some families say that informal interviews with their ill family member have provided both a rich experience in the present and a lasting legacy for others to enjoy. From the creation of these life-affirming narratives the ill person derives the meaning of death and dying. (See Appendix C for a good list of questions from the 2009 study of preparation and life completion, as referenced above.)

The theories mentioned above are *psychospiritual* in nature. They go beyond body and mind into the spiritual territory of meaning and transcendence. What does a psychospiritual approach to the end of life look like?

The psychospiritual approach utilizes both traditional psychological theories of human growth and a spiritual approach to support the individual on their particular journey. This spiritual approach recognizes and accesses higher consciousness using tools such as meditation, imagery, metaphor, visualization, creative arts, awareness, intuition and inner attunement, all of which are used in the pursuit of understanding (Di Vilio, 2017).

The tools for accessing higher consciousness are made for the exploration of the mythos qualities of mystery and meaning. They require a different kind of language that goes beyond medical science and speaks instead to inner wisdom and the quality of *not-knowing*. This language tells stories that are often missing from conversations about end-of-life and medical decision-making.

Some narratives are related in the language of poetry, myth, and archetype. These stories shed a different light on the facts of our dying. They give us a different perspective, a wider angle. They serve to connect us to our common humanity and to the universal story of living and dying. They offer non-rational, mythic cues for locating ourselves amidst uncertainty and hard times. For example, let's consider this poem by David Wagoner (1999).

Lost

Stand still. The trees ahead and the bushes beside you
Are not lost. Wherever you are is called Here,
And you must treat it as a powerful stranger,
Must ask permission to know it and be known.
The forest breathes. Listen. It answers.
I have made this place around you;
If you leave it you may come back again, saying Here.
No two trees are the same to Raven.
No two branches are the same to Wren.
If what a tree or a bush does is lost on you,
You are surely lost. Stand still. The forest knows
Where you are. You must let it find you.

From this poem we intuit that humans should not expect to easily or habitually find our way through this territory – we need to pay close attention to the world around us. The poem is asking us to stop, listen, and be in silence. It also recognizes that becoming lost is part of life.

Dark places, often represented in myths and fairy tales as a deep forest, are where people become lost and disoriented. When experiencing serious illness, this in-between phase "in the forest" is where many of us experience isolation, anxiety, and brokenness. We are separated from home and all that is familiar, but it's not yet clear where we're going. The idea of the *hero's journey*, a story line running through many fairy tales and Greek myth, was popularized by the scholar Joseph Campbell in his book, *Hero With a Thousand Faces*. The myth tells of tasks and trials we must undertake in unfamiliar places, with gifts of wisdom (lessons learned) at the end of each. A key figure or guide, often supernatural, usually helps us at key moments of danger or crisis. It turns out that we can find *value* in this dark and unfamiliar place. We experience elements of life review, the healing of old wounds, deeper love, forgiveness, gratitude, kindness, and wisdom. We are challenged as never before, find courage along the way, and follow the path out of the forest (Bronzite, 2017). This journey takes us back home and yet, as familiar as this place may be, we re-enter it as someone fundamentally changed.

IT MAY BE THAT WHEN WE NO LONGER KNOW WHAT TO DO THAT WE HAVE COME TO OUR REAL WORK AND THAT WHEN WE NO LONGER KNOW WHICH WAY TO GO WE HAVE BEGUN OUR REAL JOURNEY. THE MIND THAT IS NOT BAFFLED IS NOT EMPLOYED. THE IMPEDED STREAM IS THE ONE THAT SINGS.
–Wendell Berry, Standing by Words

This archetypal motif of a *journey* recurs in formal studies of dreams, myths, rites of passage, and spirituality, as well as in literature and art. The journey involves travel from the present to another place, and sometimes back again. For many of us who have worked in end-of-life care, this metaphor of a *journey* or *trip* is often used by dying people who experience near-death or "nearing-death" awareness. Maggie Callanan and Patricia Kelly, two pioneers in hospice nursing, have researched the states of awareness and consciousness in the dying. In their book *Final Gifts* (1992), they note that similar patterns of symbolic language are expressed regardless of the person's age, gender, ethnicity, race, medications, type of illness, or religious beliefs. Their extensive data point to two main categories of messages: what people were *experiencing* (for example, being in the presence of someone no longer alive who guides them, or the need to prepare for a trip), or what they *needed* so death could be peaceful, such as reconciliation of relationship.

The universality of these experiences is fascinating, drawing common themes from a diversity of times, places, and people. How do we prepare for the journey at end of life? What do we need to find our way through these unfamiliar, sometimes frightening places?

THERE'S A THREAD YOU FOLLOW. IT GOES AMONG THINGS THAT CHANGE. BUT IT DOESN'T CHANGE.

In his poem *The Way It Is*, William Stafford refers to the steadfast presence of a "thread" of continuity. It's possible for people with serious illness to become disoriented, losing track of the thread of *what matters most*. Many times hospice patients and families say that they regret spending their last months tied to a cycle of treatments and hospitalizations, missing out on the chance to be with family or enjoying simple time at home. This regret also expresses a recognition that they didn't explore other options – they were putting all their energies into not *dying*. How might the health care team around them have supported them to consider alternatives?

Reflective practices and conversations, ideally undertaken long before the end of life, are one means of holding onto and following Stafford's thread. The poet speaks to us as a wise elder as he ends his poem:

NOTHING YOU DO CAN STOP TIME'S UNFOLDING
YOU DON'T EVER LET GO OF THE THREAD.

Stu Farber, a pioneer of palliative medicine, used this thread in Stafford's poem to describe his experience of navigating end-stage leukemia. He writes:

> The clinicians who treated me have good hearts, care deeply, but possess little or no knowledge of my thread. My thread is the narrative I use to make sense of my life. It is longitudinal, non-linear, emotional, filled with contradictions, and integrates my life experiences into a coherent whole. It is within the values and meanings of my story that treatment decisions are made. What contributes to meaning and quality is not about living longer but living a life that is consistent with my thread (2015).

I've witnessed over the years that when people take time to reflect, prepare, and communicate a plan ahead of time for the last part of their lives, a *shift* happens. They are more able to let "what matters most" be their guide – their thread – through the challenging path of aging and advanced illness. They avoid the unnecessary suffering – for themselves and their families – that often results when difficult decisions are made in crisis as our bodies are dying. And they wake up to the preciousness of life – often with renewed purpose and gratitude.

There is still much that is unknown and mysterious in the process of dying. A focus on medical diagnosis, treatment, and prognosis isn't enough to tell the story. As nurse coaches, we might benefit from a different kind of conversation to illuminate the unfamiliar journey through the last part of life, a different context to hold this complex experience. Perhaps a fresh perspective can help us imagine the challenges of illness and dying differently. The provocative end-of-life thought-leader Stephen Jenkinson speaks to the experience of many Americans who come into their dying time as if *blindsided* by the news. We are surprised and caught unaware, despite the evidence of our failing bodies, old age, and medical treatments that are no longer effective. The possibility of dying is often resisted by people as they near the end of their lives. In exploring this disconnection from the natural order of living and dying, Jenkinson asks these key questions: "How do you find out where in your life you are? Where are you in the arc of your days?" (2016).

An exploration of the developmental stages of human life as we age, live with advanced illness, and die is one way to find ourselves in the "arc of our days." Our stories are complex – they contain tasks of development, life review, discovery of purpose, spiritual exploration, and experiences of healing and wellbeing. We move from one place to another through rites of passage, mythic trials, and states of consciousness. Knowing our own story – and how other humans have navigated the end of their lives – has the potential to bring meaning and value into these times of great transition.

New Wave of Innovation

Does this exploration of the human story change the conversation about end-of-life care? It may be an important factor in the cultural shift we're witnessing. A second wave of innovation and fresh conversations about the place of dying is already happening, with new models emerging for how we talk about dying, how we care for people at end of life, how we more consciously prepare for death, and how we create after-death practices. These innovative models are arising at the leading edge of hospice and palliative care, institutions that, 40 years ago, were the new models and "disruptors" of their time. Today's innovative projects are intentional in their desire to bring the subjects of death and dying further into the open. Nurse coaching – and coaching conversations – are part of that movement forward.

There is a generational piece to this new wave of change, with Baby Boomers and Millennials leading the way. Baby Boomers have been awakened to the realities of modern dying and caregiving through their parents' (and their own) experiences. They are redefining aging and retirement for themselves just as they did for earlier stages of their lives. The younger generation, which is fueling much of the freshest thinking about the place of death in our culture, brings a certain counter-cultural perspective and communitarian approach to our societal conversation. Furthermore, their engagement with social media has exposed them to a variety of information about death and dying that wouldn't have been available even a few years ago. This second wave might be seen as a recalibration, a "course correction" yet again to address the bigger picture of the place and significance of death in our lives.

Many innovative projects and initiatives now emerging are a healthy response to imbalances in and unhealthy facets of our experience of aging and dying. They have emerged naturally and organically out of a deep desire for a different model for the end of life.

As someone who coaches others in the art of possibilities, you are part of this changing culture. I encourage you to stay curious and engaged with this unfolding story. Below are some examples of innovations that are moving into the mainstream of our culture. Each example falls into a category of innovation and is placed in the context of what challenges it addresses and what purpose it might serve. Additional examples and links can be found in *Appendix A.*

Category of Innovation	Challenges Addressed	Specific Examples	Purposes of the Initiative
How We Age	Older people are isolated, invisible, without purpose, and not contributing to the community	• **Positive aging** This is a movement to redefine aging in a more positive mode with a focus on strength, resilience, and full engagement with life as we age. • **Conscious aging** Similar to positive aging, this approach brings in practices from spirituality and mindfulness for a deeper focus on wisdom and purpose in the last third of our lives. • **"Encore" careers** For some, it's a chance to have a second career, doing more meaningful work. For others, it's a way to have purpose and stay engaged as an older adult in either volunteer or paid capacity. • **Multigenerational learning** Whether in schools, neighborhoods or workplaces, older adults benefit from teaching and learning in an intentional multigenerational environment. • **Innovative housing options** A growing number of affordable and community- oriented housing and living options are available: Cohousing, house sharing, aging-in-place communities, housing cooperatives, affinity retirement communities, and "tiny houses." (https://bit.ly/2JL9Kyh)	Creating opportunities for elders to share their life skills and wisdom with others. Keeping elders engaged in their communities and with younger generations.

Category of Innovation	Challenges Addressed	Specific Examples	Purposes of the Initiative
How we talk about death and dying	Death is a taboo subject. Death is a failure of medicine. Many people don't know how to start these conversations.	**• Death cafes** Started in Europe in 2004, these are informal discussion groups within communities around the world to talk about death informally among strangers – over food and drink. https://deathcafe.com **• The Conversation Project** This organization provides conversation "starter kits" for people wishing to talk more openly about their preferences for end-of-life care. https://bit.ly/2lvqvkY **• Let's Have Dinner and Talk About Death** This website provides user-friendly materials to organize a dinner party for friends, family, or strangers with the express purpose of talking about death and dying in a social setting. Included are e-mail invitation, conversation prompts, and tips for a successful experience. https://deathoverdinner.org/ **• Social media stories** Stories about living with serious illness, dying, caregiving, and funerals are being shared in multiple forms – blogs, Facebook posts, Twitter messages, and e-mail messages. For example, Scott Simon tweets about his mother's dying, https://n.pr/2O1kXsQ); and country singer Rory Feek chronicles his wife Joey's illness and dying. https://on.today.com/2CfZkAu **• "Get your shit together" website** Chanel Reynolds created this website after her young husband died unexpectedly and she was completely unprepared. Easy-to-use resources cover legal and financial forms and planning, insurance, and end-of- life wishes. https://www.gyst.com	Topics of serious illness, death & dying can be normalized and discussed out in the open.

Category of Innovation	Challenges Addressed	Specific Examples	Purposes of the Initiative
How we make medical decisions	The imperative of the medical model is to not die. Medical decisions are made at the last minute, and in times of crisis. People named as medical power of attorney may not be clear about the other person's wishes.	**• 5 Wishes** This booklet supports conversations about advance care planning. The living will and power of attorney forms, as well as three other wishes for end-of-life care (comfort, how to be treated, and what loved ones should know)are legally valid in most states. https://agingwithdignity.org **• POLST/MOLST forms** Physician (or Medical) Orders for Life-Sustaining Treatments are completed by a physician, summarize a person's end-of-life wishes, and give medical orders for emergency health care professionals to follow. It goes into the person's medical record and is portable. (Not all states have these forms available.) https://bit.ly/2Ux25og **• Stanford Letter Project** This website provides letter templates to make it easier to communicate end-of-life wishes and decisions, including a "What matters most" letter, a letter project on advance directives, and a "friends and family" letter. https://stan.md/2J8u4cE **• "The right to die" movement** Compassion & Choices is the oldest, largest, and most active organization advocating for expanding options through the end of life. It focuses on medical aid for dying, physician-assisted suicide, and the right for individuals to end their own lives. https://bit.ly/1pfYJ1C	Decisions about treatment and end-of-life wishes can be discussed throughout the course of illness, and shared with significant family members. Decisions can be based on what matters most to the individual.

Category of Innovation	Challenges Addressed	Specific Examples	Purposes of the Initiative
How we experience the time of dying	Individuals and their families are isolated, overwhelmed, and fearful.	**• Death doulas** Based on the role of birth doulas, death doulas (also called end-of-life doulas or death midwives) sit vigil with a dying person, support the family, and may also assist with paperwork and legacy projects. The role is undefined and unregulated at this point, and training exists for lay people and health professionals alike... National End-of-Life Doula Alliance (https://bit.ly/2T1efnN) **• Living wakes** A funeral or memorial service may be held while the dying person is still living, so they can be part of it. Also called a "living funeral," "awake wake," or "pre-death ceremonial farewell," these events can be organized by family and friends, a death planner, or a funeral home. **• Comfort Care Homes** This new model for caring for dying people draws on the help of volunteers and nurses and provides care in a home setting at no cost to patient or family. It meets the needs of hospice patients who don't have a home, can't afford nursing facilities, or may have limited housing options. Also called social hospice homes. **• Conscious dying** This perspective brings together healing, wisdom traditions, and spiritual awakening for the time of dying. Many resources are available to prepare, support, and guide people: classes, training programs, books, podcasts, and more. Resources often come from Hindu, Buddhist, or esoteric Christian roots, as well as current consciousness studies that include research into topics such as near-death experiences and the use of psilocybin for death anxiety.	The last part of life has the potential to be a time of healing, life review, and closure for an individual and a family. It is a vital stage of life that has its own purpose and meaning.

Category of Innovation	Challenges Addressed	Specific Examples	Purposes of the Initiative
After- death care	After-death care is only done by funeral professionals, immediately after death. Funeral arrangements are expensive, and burial options are limited.	**• Home funerals** There is a growing movement for do-it-yourself home funerals including hands-on preparation of the body, vigil/visitation, and simple burials. Often coordinated by a death midwife or death planner, this is part of the larger movement of "natural death care" that strives to bring dying and burials closer to what they were like in the past, particularly in terms of simplicity and community participation. **• Green burials** So-called green or natural burials are an environmentally friendly alternative to normal funeral procedures such as embalming and heavy caskets. These practices feature non-toxic and biodegradable materials. **• Non-traditional millennial morticians** A younger generation of morticians and funeral directors are more open to non-traditional funeral and burial practices. For example, Caitlin Doughty founded The Order of the Good Death, a collaborative project of progressive after-death care that includes Katrina Spade of the Urban Death Project and Jae Rhim Lee of the Infinity Burial Suit/ Mushroom Death Suit. These thought-leaders play a part in the death-positive movement.	Some people find it meaningful and rewarding to be part of the long-time custom of cleaning and dressing the body after death—as well as holding the funeral at home. Other people are conscious of the negative environmental impact of standard funeral preparations.

Reflective Practices

1. Have you ever been to a death café (deathcafe.com)? If so, what surprised you about it? If you are unable to find one in your area to visit, what intrigues you about the idea?

2. Do you remember a time when you were in a "dark place in the forest" in your life, when you felt lost and no longer knew what to do or where to go? What was the turning point in finding your way out?

3. What is one thread in your life that you don't ever want to let go of? How do you recognize it? How will you keep a hold of it in the months and years ahead?

4. Imagine you have six months to live.

- Make a list of who and what you value most.

- From that list, identify what are your priorities are.

- Who is on the team that will help you through the last six months?

- Of the people you value most, is there anything you need to say that hasn't been said already?

- How do you want to spend your time?

- What experiences do you want to have?

- Where do you want to be during that time?

- What practical things – paperwork, legal business, etc. –need to be done?

- What do you want to do with your favorite or prized possessions?

- How do you want to say goodbye to people you care about?

- What life wisdom or legacy do you want to leave behind? For whom?

What if you didn't wait until you had months to live, but lived that way now? What on the list would be the first thing you'd do?

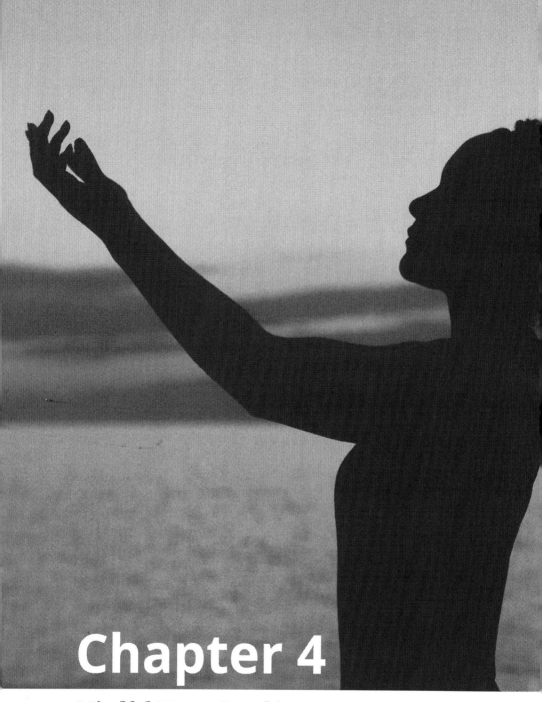

Chapter 4

Mindful Nurse Coaching:
Resilience and Self-care

Mindful Nurse Coaching: Resilience and Self-care

Quality of life isn't just a goal for people at the end of their lives. Nor is wellbeing only for patients and their families. In order for nurse coaching to be sustainable and enjoyable, we need to prioritize quality of life and wellbeing for *ourselves* as well. And we need to cultivate our capacity to be with suffering, both our own and others.'

Nurse coach self-development is a process where we take personal responsibility for our growth, development, and self-care. It is an essential part of being a healthy and resilient nurse coach. The importance of self-care is a frequent topic in health care wellness programs, as there's much evidence that professional caregivers are often better at taking care of others than they are at taking care of themselves. As the wellness nurse for a large hospice organization, I frequently saw the consequences of chronic stress and fatigue on staff members, including an increase in absenteeism, physical illness, low morale, and workplace injury.

Wellness initiatives are often short-term and based on an education model – the assumption is that if people are given encouragement and health promotion materials, they are bound to practice better self-care. However, I have observed over many years that some of the most effective and long-lasting methods of cultivating consistent self-care and wellbeing for nurses are related to the practices of *mindfulness* and *coaching*.

Self-care is manifested in the practices and habits we intentionally choose as the means to the end goal of wellbeing and balance. These practices and habits are behavior-based and active – they are not simply hopes and ideas. The coaching model is very effective in guiding us to make behavior changes that lead to regular self-care practices that are based on our priorities and what matters most. We build on our strengths and our motivation to form a plan that is realistic and achievable. We maintain self-care real by having a clear goal, breaking it down into manageable action steps, and then taking one step forward at a time.

What we seek to build through self-care is *resiliency* – a capacity to cope with stress and adversity. Research from the field of positive psychology shows us that resiliency is not a personality trait, but rather a skill that can be learned and encouraged. The American Psychological Association defines resilience as "the human ability to adapt in the face of tragedy, trauma, adversity, hardship, and ongoing significant life stressors." As nurses we had to learn to adapt and cope with many situations of significant human pain and suffering. Our capacity to be with suffering – to be empathic and caring towards others – is a real strength. However, without steady self-care practices this capacity can diminish, and we may begin to feel the drain of compassion fatigue and burnout.

Compassion fatigue is the cumulative effect of witnessing illness, loss, and death on a regular basis. It also reflects the cumulative grief we have carried, sometimes unknowingly, for years. This strain and weariness evolves over time and takes a toll on our whole being – body, mind, and spirit.

For health professionals, compassion fatigue arises when providers have close interpersonal contact with a suffering patient and their emotional boundaries become blurred to the point that the caregiver unconsciously assimilates the distress experienced by the patient (Bush, 2009).

As a result of our frequent and close connections with patients and families, nurses are particularly vulnerable to compassion fatigue. Perhaps we never learned solid strategies for communicating with patients and families facing heightened stress or complex emotional needs. We may not have found healthy role models for maintaining boundaries, reframing difficult situations, or managing conflict.

Signs and symptoms of compassion fatigue and burnout – increased irritability, anger, anxiety, depression, difficulty concentrating, fatigue, somatic complaints, sleep disturbances, emotional withdrawal, and absenteeism – may appear similar, but their etiology and outcomes are different. *Compassion fatigue* comes directly from empathically caring for suffering and traumatized people. Its advent is often more sudden, while burnout is gradual and takes place over time. *Burnout* is more a response to work or environmental stressors such as staffing, workload, or management decisions. The outcome of compassion fatigue is an imbalance of empathy and objectivity; burnout leads to decreased empathy and withdrawal.

Moral distress is another layer of professional strain that may be experienced when the nurse considers the care being provided as ethically challenging or medically inappropriate. More common in acute care settings when cure is still the focus, this distress may also arise in palliative settings. Cynda Rushton, an internationally known nurse ethicist, encourages us to reflect on the practice of *moral resilience*, which leads to increased *moral courage*. With courage and clarity, we are more likely to find our voice and speak out. We build this resilience through reflective practices such as:

- knowing who we are as a person and what we stand for

- exploring our own values and beliefs conscientiously

- being responsive and flexible in complex ethical situations (2016).

Compassion and the *ability to be with suffering* are two essential skills for nurse coaches to cultivate. When cultivating compassion, we engage in a deliberate process of developing the qualities and skills of compassion. We go beyond the habitual belief supported by our culture that suffering hurts, and our goal should be to avoid it whenever possible. Instead we ask, "What would it take to create a different relationship with our suffering?" How might we move towards, rather than away from, our pain and suffering? We can start by looking at all the ways we avoid suffering – and today we have so many more creative ways to distract ourselves from our suffering! We can learn about and then practice ways to open ourselves to our own and others' broken-heartedness without feeling despair or becoming overwhelmed. It starts with sitting still and learning to be in the present moment or, as they say in humorous Buddhist circles, "Sit. Stay. Heal."

When we stay present and engaged with very ill and dying people, we create a relationship of authenticity and connection that deepens the possibilities for healing on a psychospiritual level. To be present is to *be* in the *present*. There is a qualitatively different feel when someone is with me – fully present – as compared to someone whose mind seems distracted and distant. In coaching we call that *therapeutic presence* – being physically, emotionally, cognitively, and spiritually present with another person. When we can be with suffering in the present moment, there is no past or future to distract our minds. There is only what is passing through our body, mind, and spirit in that particular moment. Moment by moment, we can move through painful, difficult feelings. When we engage in mindful practices, we are "paying attention on purpose" to body, mind, and spirit.

A focus on our breathing is a natural way for us to pay attention to what is happening in this moment, right now. We follow the breath in, and we follow it out. We may notice how it moves through our nostrils, the rise and fall of our chest or belly. By noticing what is happening in the moment, we are better able to recalibrate thoughts and feelings, to see them as moving through us like mini-weather patterns. Here, a storm…there, blue sky…over there, not much happening. There is no expectation of how things should be, or should have been. That expectation is part of our suffering, this resistance to what *is*. As we practice this awareness of ourselves in the present moment, we increase our capacity for being present with others.

Cultivating compassionate presence helps the difficult work of being with seriously ill and dying people become more *sustainable*. Most of those who feel called to this work want to be able to do it for a long time. Without attention to the health of our bodies, hearts, and spirits, however, there is a greater likelihood of burnout or compassion fatigue over time. Frank Ostaseski spoke to healthcare workers in a 2011 interview.

> The word "compassion" means literally to "suffer with others."
> It's the little word "with" in the middle which is so important,
> because it implies a certain kind of intimacy, a willingness to "be
> with." This doesn't mean that we have to get lost in the suffering
> of others. We have to be able to build an empathetic bridge from
> our own experience to theirs. So if we never turn toward our own
> suffering – and healthcare workers are generally encouraged
> not to — we are increasingly unable to make that bridge.

It is likely most of us didn't learn these skills in our nursing training and education. However, many of us have intuitively moved in these directions, without knowing that we could more intentionally develop this practice. Today there are many more resources available for studying and developing mindful, compassionate practices – they can be found online, in books and magazines, through apps on our phones, or in research studies in professional journals. Barbara Dossey and Cynda Rushton, international nurse thought-leaders who teach contemplative practices for compassionate end-of-life care to nurses and others, write:

> Being with dying people is an integral part of nursing, yet
> many nurses feel unprepared to accompany people through the
> process of dying. Today's fast-paced healthcare environment
> conditions us to view death as a physiologic event, not as the
> sacred passage of a life, and as a failure, not as part of the human
> life cycle. To create a safe passage for patients and families, we
> need a holistic approach and skills that allow us to witness the
> dying process with compassion and strength (2007).

Dossey and Rushton invite us to imagine the development of compassionate presence as an integration of three parts: *not knowing*, *bearing witness*, and *acting compassionately.* "Not knowing" is probably an uncomfortable place for most of us working in health care. Our competence, use of scientific data, and expertise is not only expected but evaluated on a regular basis. A "not knowing" state of mind requires an awareness of – and then a letting go of – fixed ideas about ourselves and the world around us. For example, when we're working with a seriously ill person, the more we let go of our ideas about what they should do next, what treatments they should or shouldn't do, or what the outcome of our conversation should be, the more opportunity there is to ask the questions that lead that person to their *own* inner wisdom and answers.

Bearing witness to suffering is central to working with people as a healthcare professional. We witness suffering on all levels, be it physical, emotional, psychological, spiritual, economic, ethical, or community-wide. A key practice that helps prevent burnout is the practice of *being present* with *what is.* Being present doesn't just happen – it takes practice to develop focus, stability and resilience of mind. It takes awareness of what a distracted mind feels like vs. a calmer mind. It takes practice to switch gently and without judgment from distracted thoughts to a focused, calm mind. Suffering is increased for many of us when we feel things should be different, i.e., the suffering in front of us should not be happening. The acceptance of what is in the present moment helps free us from the worries or anxieties about the past and the future.

Compassionate action is the last piece of this trio of integrated concepts that lead us towards greater compassion. The action we take is the service we provide to patients and families. This includes the practices of calmly "holding space," witnessing another's suffering, staying present and centered in times of crisis, and working from an open heart. (For a well-written description of *holding space*, see Appendix F.) These practices or actions promote healing and wholeness within a person's life. They have the potential to change the quality of mind from which we work. Such practices sustain us day after day, year after year. They also allow us to work skillfully with the suffering we encounter at end of life, whether our own of that of our patients and families.

We know that fear and anxiety are common experiences for people facing serious illness and dying. As nurse coaches become more familiar with mindfulness or awareness practices, they then integrate them into coaching sessions with patients and families. It might be a few moments of breath work at the beginning of a session, or a simple guided visualization that helps to relieve a person's anxiety. Sometimes, it's a stressed or exhausted caregiver who benefits most from a relaxation practice or mindfulness meditation. These skills of focus, detachment, and compassion are essential for anyone managing the demands of a caregiving role.

The ongoing development of self-care is enhanced both by *personal reflection* and a commitment to *taking action*. That's how these habits and practices of wellbeing take root over time in our lives. We change and transform our habits – those things we regularly and often unconsciously do, think, and feel. Stopping our habitual way of doing things allows us to be more present and to recalibrate our next steps more intentionally. Habits and practices of self-care that support wellbeing and build resiliency include:

- Work/life balance

- Eating healthfully

- Physical strength and flexibility

- Adequate rest and sleep

- Regular reflective or mindfulness practices

- Fun and laughter

- Social connections

- Purpose and meaning in life

- Practicing forgiveness and gratitude

- Asking for help and support

- Prioritizing what matters most

The coaching model offers an excellent way to make behavior changes and put new practices in place. This is another place to "walk your talk" as a nurse coach. We assess and reflect: How are things going...what's working well...where am I struggling...how might I move towards an even greater sense of wellbeing? Then we focus on creating clear, do-able steps forward towards wellbeing. Questions that might serve this purpose include:

- What do I want or hope for?

- What would I be willing to do?

- What would be a benefit of doing that?

- How important is this change to me?

The goals we set are connected directly to our wishes for greater wellbeing. They are the "what" of what matters most. They form the overall plan for where we are heading. The action steps that come out of those goals are the "how" of how we move forward. We keep the goals clear, achievable, and realistic, basing them on our own priorities and readiness to change. The first action step sets the path for what is ours to do today. In discerning how much plan and goals are in alignment with what matters most, we decide where we fall on the following scales or rulers:

> On a scale of 0-10 (10 highest), how motivated am I to change this?

> On a scale of 0-10 (10 being the most), how confident am I that I could make this change?

The ideal number would be "7" or above, as this correlates with better outcomes for change. If your number is below "7," you would likely be better off creating a more achievable goal that inspires greater motivation and confidence on your part.

Decisional balance is another coaching tool that may prove helpful during those times we find ourselves stuck and unable to move forward towards what matters most. This process weighs the pros and cons of changing vs. staying the same when contemplating a decision or change in behavior. We reflect on the *benefits* of not changing (staying the same), the costs of not changing, and then the costs and benefits of changing. When the benefits of change outweigh the costs, we are more likely to move forward with our plans or decisions. It's easy to see the benefit in making healthy changes in our lives, such as having more energy, more restful sleep, less pain with movement, or a clearer sense of purpose. What is often harder is to look honestly at the reasons why we choose to stay the same and avoid change. Often, we have unacknowledged reasons for keeping the status quo.

- Change may bring discomfort (as well as increased wellbeing)

- Change may alter significant relationships, as well as improve them

- Change may bring loss as well as gain.

We ask ourselves: What do I *gain* from keeping things as they are, and what do I *lose* by changing things? There are consequences when we change. If I say "yes" to one thing, what am I saying "no" to? Our beliefs often operate on a subconscious level, but they can still play a powerful role in either helping us or tripping us up. We may be holding onto old, familiar habits because we don't want to experience the loss involved in moving forward.

Reflecting on our own beliefs and experiences increases our awareness, which in turn builds our skills as reflective practitioners. We make choices – and take action – out of that awareness. Awareness and choice are key building blocks of integrative nurse coaching.

> The ultimate outcome of caring for self is to become more fully human, to understand what it means to be a person within the world, and to act on the increased understanding. (Lauterbach, 1996)

At the heart of this process of mindful nurse coaching is a *shift* towards change and growth. This shift involves taking more responsibility for our own health and wellbeing, experiencing greater quality of life, being more compassionately present in the world, and creating a more coherent view of we might live successfully to the end of our life. As Richard Moss writes,

> Surrendering to change is always a leap of faith. For something new to enter your life, you have to let go of the past and join your immediate experience right now. The key is less in what you do than how connected you are in yourself as you do it. In life there is no predetermined path you should or have to walk; you lay down the path by how you take each step. This is one of life's greatest truths.

Every journey – whether our own or those we are fortunate to serve as nurse coaches – starts with a single step forward. Be well as you step forward on your path.

Reflective Practices:

1. When you start to feel emotional or spiritual pain, what is your usual response? What do you do that serves you well in managing pain and suffering? What kinds of things do you use to numb yourself from pain and suffering?

2. Bring to mind something you've been struggling to change in your health habits – something that would make you feel more healthy, balanced, or energized. What are the reasons to change? What are the benefits of not changing, keeping things as they are? Which one of these is stronger in you right now?

If the desire to change is stronger, consider on a scale of 1-1, how motivated you are to make this change. On a scale of 1-10, how confident are you that you can move forward with this change?

What's one thing you could do today towards reaching that goal?

3. Four Things That Matter Most. Ira Byock writes that four simple phrases— "Please forgive me," "I forgive you," "Thank you," and "I love you"—carry great power to mend and nurture our relationships and inner lives, especially in the last part of our lives. Next to the phrase below, write the name of a person (or persons) you would like to say this to.

Please forgive me, _____

I forgive you, _____

I love you, _____

Thank you, _____

Is there anything else you would like say to these people? Might you say this to some of these people now? Or soon?

4. Sometimes we are not kind, compassionate, or forgiving with ourselves. Make a list of the ways you *have* been kind and compassionate with yourself over the past few weeks, whether through thoughts, words, or actions. Which of these are you willing to increase for the next week?

If you have found these reflective practices helpful or insightful, consider trying others from the list in *Appendix D*. If you choose to share some with family, friends, or colleagues at an appropriate time, it may open up an interesting and meaningful conversation.

Permissions:

References

American Nurses Association. (2016). *Nurses' Roles and Responsibilities in Providing Care and Support at the End of Life* (Position Statement). http://www.nursingworld.org/MainMenuCategories/ EthicsStandards/Ethics-Position-Statements/EndofLife-PositionStatement.pdf

Austerlic, S. (2009). *Cultural humility and compassionate presence at the end of life*. Retrieved from: https://www.scu.edu/ethics/focus areas/ bioethics/resources/culturally-competent-care/from-chronic-to-critical/cultural-humilitycompassionate-presence/

Bach, V., Ploeg, J., Black, M. (2009). Nursing roles in end-of-life decision making in critical care settings. *Western Journal of Nursing Research*, 31, 4, 496-512.

Benson, W. F., Aldrich, N. (2012). Advance care planning: Ensuring your wishes are known and honored if you are unable to speak for yourself. Critical Issue Brief, *Centers for Disease Control and Prevention*. www.cdc.gov/aging

Bronzite, D. *The hero's journey: Mythic structure of Joseph Campbell's monomyth* (blog). Retrieved from website 4/15/17. http://www. movieoutline.com/articles/the-hero-journey-mythic-structure-of-joseph-campbell-monomyth.html

Bush, N. (2009, Jan.). Compassion fatigue: Are you at risk? *Oncology Nursing Forum*. 36: 1, p. 24

Byock, I. (2016). Imagining people well (chapter). *Awake at the bedside: Contemplative teachings on palliative and end-of-life care*. Wisdom Publications.

Callanan, M, Kelley, P. (1992). Final gifts: Understanding the special awareness, needs, and communications of the dying. Bantam Books.

Di Vilio, L. Introducing the psychospiritual approach. Website blog. Retrieved 4/15/17. http://www.allthingshealing.com/psycho-spiritual-healing-definition.php#.WPU3nUXyvIU

Dossey B.M., Dossey, B., Luck, S. (2015, August). Nurse coaching through a nursing lens: The theory of integrative nurse coaching. *Beginnings*.

Dossey, B. M., Luck, S., & Schaub, B. G. (2015). *Nurse coaching: Integrative approaches for health and well-being.* Miami, FL: INCA.

Farber, S. (2015). *Living every minute. Journal of Pain and Symptom Management,* 49(4), 796-800.

Flower, J. (May 2002). Excerpts from conversations with Frank Ostaseski. *Health Forum,* 1;45(3):16-8, 19-21 .https://www.mettainstitute.org/ pdfs/Work-Life-Wisdom.pdf

Gawande, A. (2014). *Being mortal: Medicine and what matters in the end.* Metropolitan Books.

Hebert, K., Moore, H., Rooney, J. (2011). The nurse advocate in end-of-life care. *The Ochsner Journal,* (11) 325-329.

Hutchinson, T. (Ed.). (2011). *Whole person care, a new paradigm for the 21st century.* Springer Press.

Institute of Medicine. (2014). *Dying in America: Improving quality and honoring individual preferences near end of life.* National Academies of Science. Washington, DC. http://nationalacademies.org/hmd/~/ media/Files/Report%20Files/2014/EOL/Key%20Findings%20 and%20Recommendations.pdf

Jenkinson, S. (2015). *Die wise: A manifesto for sanity and soul.* North Atlantic Books.

Kubler-Ross, E. (1969). *On death and dying: What the dying have to teach doctors, nurses, clergy and their own families.* N.Y.: Macmillan Publishing Co.

Lauterbach, S. S., Becker, P. H. (1996, Jan.). *Caring for self: Becoming a self-reflective nurse, Holistic Nursing Practice.*

Levine, S. (1982). *Who dies?: An investigation of conscious living and conscious dying* Garden City, N.Y.: Anchor Press/Doubleday.

Meade, M. (2016). *Why myth, why now?* Mosaic Voices podcast, Living Myth, Episode 1.

Meier, E. A., Gallegos, J. V., Montross Thomas, L. P., et al. (2016). Defining a good death (successful dying): Literature review and a call for research and public dialogue. *Journal of Geriatric Psychiatry.*24, 4, 261-271.

Murray, S, Kendall, M., et al. (2005). Illness trajectories and palliative care, *BMJ*.

Ostaseski, F. (2008, April). Simple human kindness. *CIIS Public Programs Newsletter*.

Peereboom, K., Coyle, N. (2012). Facilitating goals-of-care discussions for patients with life-limiting disease – communication strategies for nurses. *Journal of Hospice and Palliative Nursing*, 14, 4, 251-258.

Pollak, K. I., Childers, J. W., Arnold, R. M. (2011). Applying motivational interviewing techniques to palliative care communication. *Journal of Palliative Medicine*, (14)5, 587-592.

Psychology Today website. *All about wisdom* (Blog). https://www.psychologytoday.com/basics/wisdom

Rushton, C. (2016). Moral resilience: A capacity for navigating moral distress in critical care. *AACN Advanced Critical Care*. 27:1, 111-119

Rushton, C., Halifax, J., Dossey, B. (2007). Being with dying: contemplative practices for compassionate end-of-life care. *American Nurse Today*, 2, 9, 16-18.

Sanders, J. (2015). *The Serious Illness Care Program: Considering health literacy for a scalable intervention to improve serious illness care* (PowerPoint presentation). http://www.nationalacademies.org/hmd/~/media/Files/Activity%20Files/PublicHealth/HealthLiteracy/July%202015%20PPTs/Justin%20Sanders.pdf

Steinhauser, K. E., Alexander, S., Byock, I., et al. (2009). Seriously ill patients' discussions of preparation and life completion: An intervention to assist with transition at end of life. *Palliative and Supportive Care*, 7, 393-404.

Thacker, K. (2008). Nurses' advocacy behaviors in end-of-life nursing care. *Nursing Ethics*, (15)2, 174-183.

Yadav, K. N., Gabler, N. B., Cooney, E., et al. (2017). Approximately one in three US adults completes any type of advance directive for end-of-life care. *Health Affairs*, 36, 7, 1252-1257.

Appendices

Appendix A
Additional Innovative End-of-Life Projects

How we age

- Music & memory programs: https://bit.ly/2UzTO2W

- Mindfulness & neural plasticity (new research on the mind & cognition) https://bit.ly/2HuhZfh

- TED talk on Alzheimer's & improv: https://bit.ly/2J839Og

How we make decisions about end of life

- Intentional end of life: Physician-assisted suicide: https://bit.ly/1pfYJ1C

- Voluntarily stopping eating & drinking (VSED): https://nyti.ms/2T1y5zf

How we talk about death & dying

- "My Gift of Grace" cards: http://mygiftofgrace.com

- The "Go Wish" card game: http://www.gowish.org

- Legacy work (https://bit.ly/2v2YvbA) – ethical wills, creative projects, life stories written or recorded (https://bit.ly/2TQWV9H)

- Pop-up death salon: https://bit.ly/2F73lZM

- Research at NYU and JHU on psychedelics & severe death anxiety: https://bit.ly/2gOCq60

- "We Croak" app (https://apple.co/2WoV5jZ) – Receive (5) daily reminders of your mortality via quotes

End-of-Life projects

- Before I Die art project: https://beforeidieproject.com

- Wake Up to Dying project: www.wakeuptodyingproject.org/

- Redesigning Death movement: www.redeath.org

- Shared Death Experience: www.sharedcrossing.com

- End Of Life University, Dr. Karen Wyatt: www.eoluniversity.com

- Re-designing death – DIY projects: https://bit.ly/2F9tlE1

- Legacy projects: https://bit.ly/2HidvZS

- Reimagine EOL: https://letsreimagine.org/

Appendix B
Useful Language in Goals-of-Care Discussions

Assess understanding of diagnosis/prognosis

- How are things going?
- What is your understanding of what has happened?
- What have the doctors told you about your condition?
- What information do you need right now?

Exploratory questions

- Tell me more...
- Can you explain what you mean?
- Can you tell me what you're worried about?
- You said you were worried about going home. Tell me more...
- How can I be of help to you?

Assess patient's support systems and coping mechanisms

- Is this the most stressful time of your life?
- How have you handled stress in the past?
- Where are you getting your support?
- What/who is helping you the most?
- How does your family communicate with each other?
- Can you anticipate any potential areas of concern for the family?
- Is there anyone you rely on to help you make important decisions?
- Who are the important people to be at a family meeting?

Define the patient's goals of care

- What do you hope for most in the next few months?
- What are your goals?
- What is important to you right now?
- Is there anything you are afraid of?

Pertinent questions to ask family members when the patient is not able to make his/her own healthcare decisions

- Tell me about your loved one.

- Tell me about his/her life so I can learn a little about him/her as a person.

- What was important to him/her?

- Did he/she ever discuss what would be important to him/her at end of life from a quality-of-life point of view?

- Did he/she discuss what sort of care he/she would want or would not want (e.g., tube feedings, attempted resuscitation, ventilator support) if he/she was terminally ill?

From the article "Facilitating goals-of-care discussions for patients with life-limiting disease: Communication strategies for nurses." (https://bit.ly/2ToYJIs) Karen Peereboom and Nessa Coyle, *Journal of Hospice and Palliative Nursing*, June 2012

Also see The Serious Illness Conversation Guide (Ariadne Labs) https://bit.ly/2prGCjU

The **End-of-Life Nursing Education Consortium (ELNEC)** project is a national education initiative whose mission is to improve palliative care both within the United States and internationally by educating nurses on better end-of-life care. Their curriculum includes coursework on how to lead effective communication during end-of-life care.

ELNEC curricula include:

- ELNEC- Core broadly outlines end-of-life care for those caring for adult patients in oncology, medical/surgical settings, hospices, palliative care settings, homecare, clinics, home-based facilities, etc.

- ELNEC- Critical Care: Care for adults in critical care settings—ICU, ED, and burn units.

- ELNEC – Oncology APRN: Education and resources for oncology advanced practice nurses to prepare them to provide primary palliative care.

- ELNEC- Geriatric: Care of older adults in community-based settings including long- term care, clinics, home health and hospice.

- ELNEC- Pediatric Palliative Care: Care for neonates to adolescents

- ELNEC- APRNs: Advanced content on pain and symptom management, billing for services, starting a palliative care program, etc. This course has 2 tracks—one for adults and one for pediatrics.

Appendix C
Preparation and Completion Intervention questions: Life Story, Forgiveness, and Heritage/Legacy

Death may be inevitable, but suffering is not. Steinhauser (2009) and the researchers who conducted the study cited below were interested in addressing emotional and spiritual suffering as well as physical suffering. They found that discussion of life completion may improve important health outcomes – actually decreasing suffering and increasing quality of life – for patients at the end of life. Their model of skillful questions and deep listening is designed to help with the role transitions that occur during serious illness. The goal is to allow people to go beyond the "patient" role by integrating their whole person resources.

Session 1: Life Story

- Tell me about your life.

- What are cherished times?

- Of what are you most proud?

- If someone were to make a movie of your life, what would be important to include?

Session 2: Forgiveness

- If you were to do things again, what might you do differently?

- Are there things or times you regret?

- Is there anyone to whom you would like to offer forgiveness?

- Is there anyone from whom you would like to ask forgiveness?

- Are you at peace?

Session 3: Heritage and Legacy

- What are your most valuable lessons learned?

- What would you like to share with future generations?

- If you could choose one thing to pass on as your legacy, what would that be?

- What things would you like to accomplish?

From: *"Seriously ill patients' discussions of preparation and life completion: An intervention to assist with transition at the end of life,"* Steinhauser et al, Palliative and Supportive Care (2009), Vol. 7, pp. 393-404

Appendix D
Additional Reflective Practices

General Questions

1. What have your experiences as a nurse taught you about dying?

2. What does living well mean to you? Who would you say is someone living well?

3. What does dying well mean to you? Who would you say has died well? Is it possible?

4. When does "end of life" begin?

5. What would you say are the three biggest problems with end-of-life care in the US?

Letting Go

Think about one of the most beloved objects in your home. Find it, and take it into your hands. Look at it, think about why you love it and why it matters to you. Then think about someone you'd like to give that object to. Notice the thoughts and feelings you have about that.

- Write down why you'd like this other person to have this object. Say goodbye to the object and thank it for all the memories or values it has held for you.

- Find a good time to give both the object and your writing to the person you've chosen. Perhaps you might read your writing or find other words in the moment to share what the object has meant to you, and why you would like this person to have it now.

- Finally, be clear with this person that you have released the object. Whatever they choose to do with it is now in their hands.

Grief and loss

What are some significant losses of your life (any kind, not just death-related)? How are they still with you? How have you let them go?

Following Your Thread: Exploring Your Own Story

1. Record three key experiences/events that significantly challenge(d) you. These can be from childhood, teen years, young adult, middle adult, or older adult life, including:

- Health challenges – yours or someone close to you

- Deaths close to you

- Other significant losses

- Significant transitions or changes in your life

    –How did you respond to these events?

    –What resources did you draw upon to get through the experience?

    –What person(s) served as guide(s) for you during that time?

    –What is one key lesson you learned from each experience?

2. What has been a significant threshold period in your life, a transition between the old you and the yet-to-be you? How did you navigate that uncertain time?

3. What's your compass – your true north – that gives direction to your life? What are the qualities of your true north? How do you recognize it, or how do you know it by experience?

Exploring Your Own Beliefs, Values, and Biases

1. How do you identify yourself in terms of:

- Geographical roots

- Health status

- Race

- Ethnicity

- Gender

- Culture

- Profession or work

- Age group

- Class or status

- Urban, suburban, or rural

- Spiritual or religious beliefs (or non-belief)

- Sexual orientation

- Disability or able-bodied

- Socio-economic background

- Educational background

- Other significant identity

Which of the identifications on this list are the most significant to you?

2. What are your beliefs and customs about the time before death and after death? Do those beliefs differ from those you grew up with?

- Should a person be told they are dying?

- Who makes decisions about a dying person's care?

- Where does the dying person live before death?

- Who cares for the dying person?

- What are qualities values in a caregiver?

- What are the expectations for how the dying person – and the friends or relatives – should behave or act?

- What happens to the body after death?

- What are the rituals surrounding a person's death?

- How do people grieve? What are acceptable/unacceptable expressions of grief?

3. In your experience as a nurse, what cultural or religious beliefs about illness and dying do you find most difficult to understand? Which beliefs related to end of life are most upsetting to you? Within your own family, are there cultural or religious beliefs about illness and dying that are hard for you to understand?

4. How would you explain the importance of advance directives to someone who isn't familiar with the term, and/or has limited English skills?

Self-care

1. I feel (or felt) a great sense of wellbeing when I...

2. What renews, energizes, and/or rejuvenates you?

3. What strengths and resilience do you draw from in challenging times? What's one area you'd like to further develop?

Writing Prompts and Discussion Jumpstarters

1. Write your obituary as a poem.

2. Write a poem about what living with Alzheimer's or dementia might be like.

3. Stephen Jenkins states, "Your dying doesn't belong to you." What does that mean to you? Who does it belong to?

Creative Practices

1. Music

- Put together a playlist for life review and memories, whether yours or someone else's.

- Make a musical recording for the last weeks of your life, or a mix tape for when you're going through difficult times.

- What songs would you like played at your memorial service? Put those on a playlist.

- Get together with friends and share song(s) you'd like played at your memorial service or life celebration.

2. Photos

- Assemble a collection of your all-time favorite photos in an album or digitally.

- Choose a dozen pictures that represent different stages of your life, and make a collage or design with them.

- Think of someone to whom you would like to write a note, perhaps telling that person something you've always wanted to express, or something hard to express. Find a significant photo that reminds you of that person and make a greeting card using that image. Write your message inside and send or give it to them.

3. Collage

- Make a collage of images that bring you peace and/or joy. These could be from magazines, calendars, photographs, or greeting cards.

- Make a collage of images that represent how you would like to live the last part of your life.

4. Movies

- View movies about end of life with friends and/or family and discuss them afterwards. Some examples:

o Tuesdays with Morrie	o Babette's Feast
o Up	o Young at Heart (documentary)
o Departures	o Last Cab to Darwin
o Wit	o Griefwalker (documentary)

  https://bit.ly/2OoFbmT

Appendix E
Poems for Reflection

Below is a list of poems that may bring fresh insights as you explore change, transitions, and the meaning of dying. You may want to keep an ongoing file of poems and essays that speak to you – both for inspiration and for reflection. In my experience, the language of poetry has a way of bypassing our intellect and going into another part of our mind and heart.

"The Way It Is" by William Stafford (https://bit.ly/2NY9MBv)

"Lost" by David Waggoner (https://bit.ly/2O4vBPS)

"In Blackwater Wood" by Mary Oliver (https://bit.ly/2O4vMeo)

"Kindness" by Naomi Shihab Nye (https://bit.ly/1R4BPti)

"we are running" by Lucille Clifton (https://bit.ly/2T4ARnz)

"Today" by Jalrudin Rumi (https://bit.ly/2XQn3jY)

"The Guest House" by Jalrudin Rumi (https://bit.ly/2EV9Yxg)

"The Summer Day" by Mary Oliver (https://bit.ly/2iSJRoz)

"I Go Among Trees" by Wendell Berry (http://www.herbcraft.org/berry.html)

"When Death Comes" by Mary Oliver (https://bit.ly/2O4wpEo)

"How Could I Not Be Among You?" by Ted Rosenthal "Otherwise" by Jane Kenyon (https://bit.ly/2jBLZKb)

"Touched by an Angel" by Maya Angelou (https://bit.ly/2T1cYx1)

"The Sailing Ship" by Bishop Charles Henry Brent (https://bit.ly/2VW7ozj)

"I Will Not Die an Unlived Life" by Dawna Marcova (https://bit.ly/1WuDu1d)

"Opening Poem: Late Fragment" by Raymond Carver (https://allpoetry.com/Late-Fragment)

"The Life You Could Be Living (If You Weren't Living This One)" by Caryn Mirriam-Goldberg (https://bit.ly/2TKduUw)

Ecclesiastes 3:1-8 (The Bible - https://bit.ly/2JbpzxS)

"To a Daughter Leaving Home" by Linda Pastan (https://bit.ly/2T1QEU3)

Appendix F
Other Resources

"Holding space" by Heather Plett (https://bit.ly/2xbnz2v)

This article provides an excellent description of what it means to "hold space" for another person or persons.

BE Ready Checklist (https://bit.ly/2HhFM2Y)

This checklist by hospice physician Dr. Karen Wyatt is a practical listing of the things that can be included in the directive to "get your affairs in order." It's likely that people you work with will find this helpful.

"How not to say the wrong thing" (https://lat.ms/2TLVXeB)

This is a practical – and humorous – article describing the "rings of kvetching" that guide you in keeping your comments appropriate and helpful.

Prepare For Your Care website (https://bit.ly/2VUnSqa)

This website offers an innovative and simplified way to fill out advance directives in both English & Spanish.

OpenIdeo.com (https://bit.ly/1XSWDt1)

This was a recent, global Request for Proposal for projects and initiatives to answer the question, "How might we reimagine the end of life for ourselves and our loved ones?"

An example of a proposal sent to the OpenIdeo.com website: Mortality coach! (https://bit.ly/2TH734K)

Podcast episodes about death and dying: Innovative podcasts from Radiolab, This American Life, Fresh Air, and others. (https://bit.ly/2J8tfk4)

TED Radio Hour (2018 NPR show) highlights the theme of "dying well" with (5) different stories. https://n.pr/2OoiH5j

Gary Malkin and Michael Stillwater CDs:

Graceful Passages: A companion for living & dying
Through words and music, this beautiful CD set offers a renewal of faith to anyone struggling with grief. The book's heartfelt words, from some of the world's greatest visionary leaders, are set to original soul-stirring music, creating an atmosphere of relaxation, insight, and healing.

Care for the Journey: Music & messages to sustain the heart of healthcare
A CD of spoken messages from leaders in compassionate care supported by original scored music -- and used by health professionals and healing practitioners as a continuing education tool and for inspirational self-renewal.

Best TED talks about end of life:
These are great to watch with other people and discuss afterwards.

ted.com/talks/timothy_ihrig_what_we_can_do_to_die_well
ted.com/talks/bj_miller_what_really_matters_at_the_end_of_life
ted.com/talks/stephen_cave_the_4_stories_we_tell_ourselves_about_death
ted.com/talks/amanda_bennett_a_heroic_narrative_for_letting_go
ted.com/talks/judy_macdonald_johnston_prepare_for_a_good_end_of_life
ted.com/talks/candy_chang_before_i_die_i_want_to
ted.com/talks/peter_saul_let_s_talk_about_dying
ted.com/talks/jae_rhim_lee
ted.com/talks/joan_halifax

Made in the USA
Las Vegas, NV
12 September 2022

55164338R00042